Impact of Disease Epidemics on the Economy: Key Considerations for Planners and Responders

Impact of Disease Epidemics on the Economy: Key Considerations for Planners and Responders

Raghu Subramaniam

SOCIETY Publishing

www.societypublishing.com

Impact of Disease Epidemics on the Economy: Key Considerations for Planners and Responders

Raghu Subramaniam

Society Publishing
224 Shoreacres Road
Burlington, ON L7L 2H2
Canada
www.societypublishing.com
Email: orders@arclereducation.com

ISBN: 978-1-77469-057-4 (Hardcover)

ABOUT THE AUTHOR

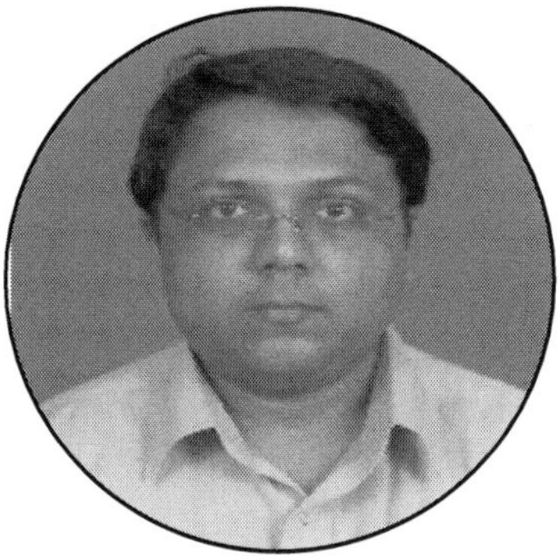

Raghu Subramaniam is based out of Chennai, Tamilnadu, and has been in the advertising space for over two decades, has managed his start-up. Raghu has been professionally writing for close to eight years now. Raghu has written extensively for some world-class medical establishments, hospitals and specialization centers. He has written technical content for a leading skincare and hair transplant clinic and has provided social media content vis-a-vis technical articles. He has also written for a Stem Cell Therapy wing of a leading hospital and has written technical content for a leading Orthopaedic Surgeon for his Endoscopic Spinal Surgery Clinic. Raghu Subramaniam has written screenplays, fictional content, essays, written and rewritten articles and scientific content especially relating to emerging technologies, electronics. He is at home with the creation of original content, as well as rewriting or enhancement of pre-written content.

TABLE OF CONTENTS

LIST OF FIGURES

LIST OF ABBREVIATIONS

AIDS	acquired immune deficiency syndrome
AP-DRG	all patient DRG
APR-DRG	all patient refined DRG
APS-DRG	all patient, severity-adjusted DRG
CDC	Centers for Disease Control and Prevention
CEPI	coalition for epidemic preparedness innovations
COPD	chronic obstructive pulmonary disease
CVD	cardiovascular disease
DALY	disability-adjusted life year
DRG	diagnosis-related group
GDP	gross domestic product
GOARN	global outbreak alert and response network
HIV	human immunodeficiency virus
IR-DRG	International-refined DRG
MERS	Middle East Respiratory Syndrome
PEPFAR	President's Emergency Plan for Aids Relief
PTSD	post-traumatic stress disorder
QALY	quality-adjusted life-year
QR	quick response
R-DRGs	refined DRGs
RSI	repetitive stress injury
SARS	severe acute respiratory syndrome
S-DRG	severity DRG
SOI	severity of illness
UNICEF	The United Nations Children's Fund
WHO	World Health Organization
YPLL	years of potential life lost

PREFACE

The year 2020 has been remarkable for many things, not the least of which is the outbreak of Coronavirus (COVID-19). This disease is airborne and has contributed to as much fear as was there during the spread of the Human Immunodeficiency Virus (HIV), which caused the Acquired Immune Deficiency Syndrome (AIDS) in its terminal stages. Another such nightmarish situation in which people are now afraid to face each other has come to pass. Different countries have reacted in different ways to COVID-19 right from those that ignored it to those that went to the other extreme of fear and literally closed down entire communities. A derogatory term, *"Covidiots"*, was coined in popular culture referring to those people who willfully ignore the "social distancing" guidelines that have been set by various administrations. One of the remarkable aspects of this outbreak has been the failure of some ostensibly wealthy nations to prepare adequately and respond to the COVID-19 crisis. This has led to many questions being raised by global preparedness to handle such an event.

This book has been conceived and set in this background. The book charts the various typologies and examples of disease outbreaks, including ones that affect animals. It highlights the impact of the epidemics on the world economy as well as the range of options that might be considered while responding to the crisis. Throughout the book, emphasis has been placed on the importance of being prepared. We live in a world which is complexly interconnected and an ever burgeoning population means that the risks of outbreaks occurring are significant. Rather than playing the blame game by trying to target the ethnicities that were initially affected by the virus and the exact geographical origins experts are calling for a unified global response that includes an understanding of the unique situations in which the victims of disease outbreaks find themselves in. It is not that the world has not felt the impact of devastating disease epidemicsDisease epidemics. The real problem has always been the extent to which the world is willing to learn lessons from the suffering of people during these events. COVID-19 has challenged the fundamental meaning various socio-economic models of disease epidemicsDisease epidemics, that are prevalent in wealthier nations.

This book is written in the spirit of having a wider conversation about disease outbreaks and their economic impact. However, considering the nature of the topics that have been covered this book would carry greater relevance to those who are involved in public health. The book is relevant to undergraduates studying a range of disciplines, including medicine, economics, social work, psychology, politics, public administration, and international affairs. The themes introduced in this book cut across categories. Hence, there is an expectation of a multi-disciplinary conceptualization in this book.

Also, the book touches on pertinent issues that arise during disease epidemicsDisease epidemics, including the social stigma that victims usually face. We already saw this happening during the HIV/AIDS crisis. The impact of that early misunderstanding of the disease are still felt today. Many people who should be getting support are not getting it, and bureaucracies sometimes stand in the way of appropriate response. Although COVID-19 is markedly different from HIV (mainly because of the mode of transmission and the speed of spread) they both share a similar economic burden of a disease epidemic that disrupts the productivity of nations. Hopefully, this book will go a long way in highlighting some of the salient issues that are associated with the medical and economic management of disease epidemicsDisease epidemics.

Chapter 1

Introduction to Disease Epidemics

CONTENTS

The opening chapter of this book explores the key aspects and conceptualizations of an epidemic disease. These interpretations are determined by the rapid spread of the disease, a wide spatial scope, the timeline of the epidemic, the populations that are most affected, and the impact of that pandemic. By the end of the chapter, the reader should have a notion of what a epidemic disease is and more importantly what does not constitute an epidemic disease, at least on the basis of modern understanding of the phenomena.

1.1. EPIDEMICS AS A RAPID SPREAD OF DISEASE

The definition of an epidemic is the rapid spread of disease to a large number of people in a given population within a short period of time (Yi-Xin and Manderson, 2005; Zadoks, 2008; Zhan, Li, Wang, Sun, Geng, Xiong, and de Hoog, 2015; Zhang, Song, Cai, and Zhou, 2008). For instance, in the case of meningococcal infections, an attack rate in excess of 15 cases per 100,000 people spread over two consecutive weeks is considered an epidemic (Weycker, Edelsberg, Oster, and Tino, 2005; Wu, Perrings, Kinzig, Collins, Minteer, and Daszak, 2017; Yach, Stuckler, and Brownell, 2006). Infectious diseases accelerating into epidemics are generally caused by several factors including a change in the ecology of the host population (Uusküla, Müürsepp, Kawai, Raag, Jürisson, and Pillsbury, 2013; Vanni, Karnon, Madan, White, Edmunds, Foss, and Legood, 2011). Common examples include increased stress or increase in the density of a vector species, a genetic change in the pathogen reservoir or the introduction of an emerging pathogen to a host population as caused by movement of pathogen or host (Tapia, 2003; Torgerson and Dowling, 2001; Torgerson, Carmona, and Bonifacino, 2000; Uddin Khan, Atanasova, Krueger, Ramirez, and Gray, 2013). Generally speaking, an epidemic occurs when host immunity to either an established pathogen or newly emerging novel pathogen is suddenly reduced below the number that constitutes the endemic equilibrium and the transmission threshold is exceeded (Suhrcke, Stuckler, Suk, Desai, Senek, McKee, and Rechel, 2011; Šumilo, Bormane, Asokliene, Vasilenko, Golovljova, Avsic-Zupanc, and Randolph, 2008). Disease epidemics Disease epidemics can have significant impacts on the politics, economics, and sociological aspects of the community (St George, 1986; Steben and Duarte-Franco, 2007; Stehr-Green and Schantz, 1987; Stuckler, 2008; Stuckler and Siegel, 2011). Figure 1.1 highlights the obvious impact of the COVID-19 pandemic on the stock market in 2020.

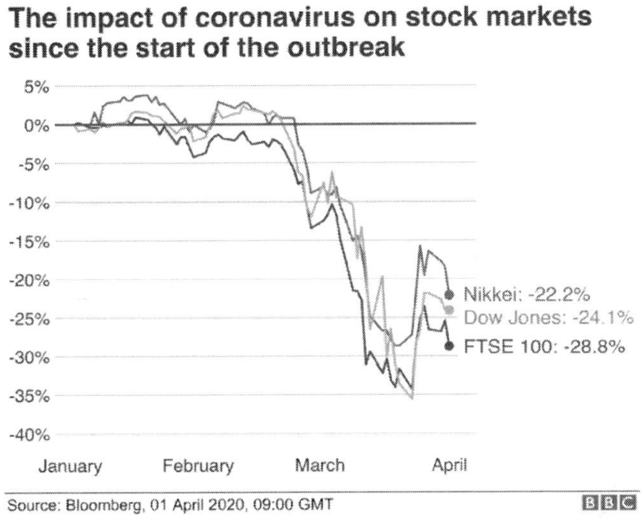

Figure 1.1. Impact of coronavirus on stock market.

Source: Bloomberg and the BBC, via the World Economic Forum.

An epidemic may be restricted to one location (Saleha, 1991; Sibert, Rigaud, Delavierre, and Labat, 2010; Skrepnek and Skrepnek, 2004; Sloane, 2009; Sockett, 1993). However, if the epidemic spreads to other countries or continents and affects a substantial number of people, it can be termed as a pandemic (Rogers, Carolin, Vaught, and Compton, 2011; Ronohardjo and Rastiko, 1982; Sachs, 2001; Sachs and Malaney, 2002). The declaration of an epidemic usually requires a good understanding of a baseline rate of incidence (Raut, 2004; Rehm, Mathers, Popova, Thavorncharoensap, Teerawattananon, and Patra, 2009; Rich and Perry, 2011). For example, epidemics for certain diseases, such as influenza, are defined as reaching an earlier defined increase in incidence above this baseline (Purevdawa, Moon, Baigalmaa, Davaajav, Smith, and Vermund, 1997; Ramesh, Malla, Raju, Sehgal, Ganguly, Mahajan, and Dilawari, 1990). Limited cases of an extremely rare disease could be classified as an epidemic, while several cases of a common disease (such as the common cold) would not be classified as an epidemic (Poundstone, Strathdee, and Celentano, 2004; Pritchett, Thilmany, and Johnson, 2005; Pugliatti, Beghi, Forsgren, Ekman, and Sobocki, 2007). An endemic can create enormous damage as a result of causing huge loss of life and of livelihood as well as tremendous financial losses (Perry and Randolph, 1999; Philipson, 2000; Philipson and Posner, 1996; Pongchaiyakul, Songpattanasilp, and Taechakraichana, 2008).

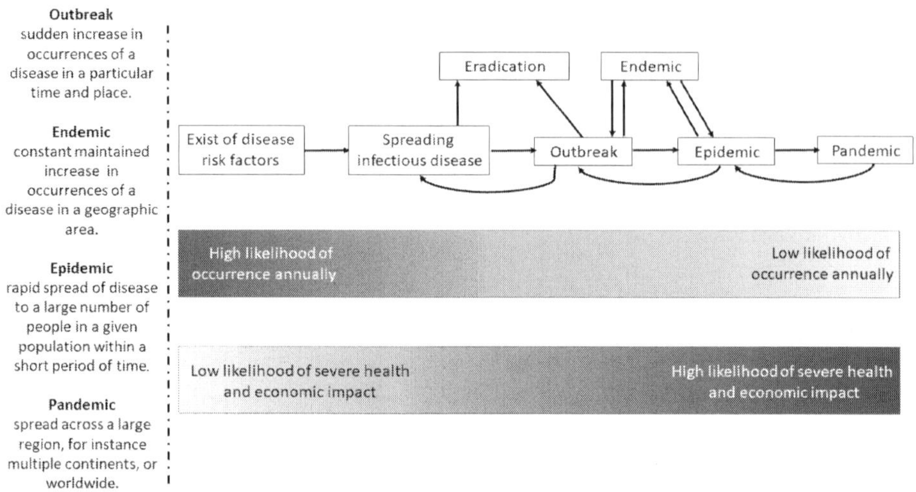

Source: By علاء (Alaa) - Own work, CC BY-SA 3.0, https://commons.wikimedia.org/w/index.php?curid=88074490

The origin of the word "epidemic" is from the Greek words epi (meaning on), and demos (meaning people), and attained first lyrical representation in Homer's Odyssey which was later incorporated in the medical field in the book Epidemics, a treatise by Hippocrates (Peckham, 2013; Perrings et al., 2002, 2014. The words "indigenous" and "endemic" were used to carry the same meaning before the usage of "epidemic" by Hippocrates (Pal, Kerorsa, Marami, and Kandi, 2020; Paterson, Otte, Slingenbergh, Wint, and Rogers, 2000; Pearce and Merletti, 2006). Thucydides' description of the Plague of Athens is considered to be one of the earliest narratives of a disease epidemic (Ozmen, Kurşun, and Ozcelik, 2005; Paarlberg, Hillberg, Lee, and Mathews, 2008; Paisley, Vraa-Andersen, Dybkjaer, Møller, Christensen, Mousing, and Agger, 1993). By the early 17th century, the terms endemic and epidemic referred to contrasting conditions of population-level disease, with the endemic condition referring to low rates of occurrence and the epidemic condition referring to widespread occurrence (Oleś, Gudowska-Nowak, and Kleczkowski, 2012; Otte, Nugent, and McLeod, 2004; Ozawa, Portnoy, Getaneh, Clark, Knoll, Bishai, and Patwardhan, 2016). The term "epidemic" has become emotionally charged, with some complaining about its use to stigmatize those that are affected by infectious diseases (Narrod, Zinsstag, and Tiongco, 2012; Nascimento and de Oliveira, 2014; O'Brien, Lahue, Caro, and Davidson, 2007).

The Centers for Disease Control and Prevention (CDC) defines epidemic broadly as the occurrence of more cases of disease, injury, or other health condition than expected in a given area, or among a specific group of persons during a particular period (Moné, Ibikounlé, Massougbodji, and Mouahid, 2010; Morand, 2004; Moro, Budke, Schantz, Vasquez, Santivanez, and Villavicencio, 2011). Usually, the cases are presumed to have a common cause or to be related to each other in some manner. The terms "epidemic" and "outbreak" have often been used interchangeably (Markos and Abdela, 2016; Martin and Shepherd, 2009; McGuinness, McGlynn, Johnson, MacIntyre, Batty, Burns, and McGinty, 2012). Researchers Manfred S. Green and colleagues propose that the term "outbreak" be restricted to smaller events, pointing out that Chambers Concise Dictionary and Stedman's Medical Dictionary acknowledge this distinction (Krieger, 2001a, b; Lemma, 1969; Liu, Maniadakis, Gray, and Rayner, 2002; López, Torné, Franco, San-Martin, Viayna, Barrull, and Perulero, 2018). There are several changes that may occur in an infectious agent that may trigger an epidemic (Kim and Goldie, 2008; Klein, Laxminarayan, Smith, and Gilligan, 2007; Klepac, Laxminarayan, and Grenfell, 2011). Some of the changes in an infectious agent that may trigger an epidemic are increased virulence, introduction into a novel setting, and changes in host susceptibility to said infectious agent (Jenkins, Baingana, Ahmad, McDaid, and Atun, 2011; Johnson, Alvarez-Pasquin, Bijl, Franco, Gaillat, Clara, and Weinke, 2015).

An epidemic disease does not necessarily have to be contagious (Howe, Häsler, and Stärk, 2013; Howe et al., 2012). For example, the term has been applied to West Nile fever and obesity as epidemics, by the World Health Organization (WHO) and other recognized institutions despite these conditions not being deemed to be highly contagious (Hart and Halden, 2020; Häsler, Howe, and Stärk, 2011; Henschke, Kamper, and Maher, 2015; Hochberg, 1992). The conditions which govern the outbreak of epidemics include infected food supplies such as contaminated drinking water and the migration of populations of certain animals, such as rats or mosquitoes, which can act as disease vectors (Foxman, 2002; Garner, Whan, Gard, and Phillips, 2001; Gayle and Hill, 2001; Gottstein, Pozio, and Nöckler, 2009). Certain epidemics are seasonal (Fenichel, 2013; Fenichel et al., 2011; Fogel, 1994). For example, whooping-cough occurs in spring, whereas measles produces two epidemics, one in winter and one in March (Espinoza, Terashima, Herrera-Velit, and Marcos, 2010; Ezzati, Vander Hoorn, Lawes, Leach, James, Lopez, and Murray, 2005). Influenza, the common cold, and other infections of the upper respiratory tract, such as sore throat, occur predominantly in the winter (Eaton and Groopman, 2013; Eckelman, Sherman, and MacNeill, 2018; Egger, 2011; Elbe, 2007; Ernst and Hay, 1994). There is another variation, both with regards to the number of people affected as well as the number who die in successive epidemics (Daily, and Ehrlich, 1996; Deogaonkar, Hutubessy, Van Der Putten, Evers, and Jit, 2012; Dorn, 1992; Ducrotoy, Bertu, Ocholi, Gusi, Bryssinckx, Welburn, and Moriyon, 2014). For instance, the severity of successive epidemics rises and falls over five or ten year periods (Chen, Li, Hsieh, Chang, Lee, Lee, and Ko, 2012; Conover, Pitt, Kessler, DuBow, and Sanborn, 1995; Crump, Murdoch, and Baker, 2001).

There are a range of typologies that are associated with pandemics (Casamassimo, Thikkurissy, Edelstein, and Maiorini, 2009; Castro, Wilson, and Bloom, 2017). In a common source outbreak epidemic, the affected individuals have an exposure to a common agent (Bwire, Munier, Ouedraogo, Heyerdahl, Komakech, Kagirita, and Makumbi, 2017; Canali, Aragrande, Angheben, Capelli, Drigo, Gobbi, and Cassini, 2020). If the exposure is singular and all of the affected individuals develop the disease over a single exposure and incubation course, it can be termed a point source outbreak (Buckley, 1984; Budke, Jiamin, Qian, and Torgerson, 2005; Bundy, Arámbulo III, and Grey, 1983; Buzby and Roberts, 2009). However, if the exposure is continuous or variable, it can be termed a continuous outbreak or intermittent outbreak, respectively (Borghol, Suderman, McArdle, Racine, Hallett, Pembrey, and Szyf, 2012; Brandes, 2008; Brown, Lipscomb, and Snyder, 2001). In a propagated outbreak, the disease spreads person-to-person (Bonds, Keenan, Rohani, and Sachs, 2010; Boni, Galvani, Wickelgren, and Malani, 2013; Bonovas and Nikolopoulos, 2012). Affected individuals may become independent reservoirs leading to further exposures (Bergevoet, Van Schaik, Veling, Backus, and Franken, 2009; Binder, 1988; Bolos, Bacarea, and Marusteri, 2011). Many epidemics will have characteristics of both common source and propagated outbreaks (Bausch and Schwarz, 2014; Bausch et al., 2001; Benner, Carabin, Sánchez-Serrano, Budke, and Carmena, 2010). This is sometimes referred to as mixed outbreak (Arredondo and Zúñiga, 2006; Backer, van Roermund, Fischer, van Asseldonk, and Bergevoet, 2015; Bartsch, Hotez, Hertenstein, Diemert, Zapf, Bottazzi, and Lee, 2016). For example, secondary person-to-person spread may occur after a common source exposure or an environmental vector spreads a zoonotic diseases agent (Armelagos, Brown, and Turner, 2005; Arokiasamy and Krishnan, 1994; Arora, 2001, 2005; Arredondo and Zúñiga, 2004).

Airborne transmission refers to the spread of infection by droplet nuclei or dust in the air (Amuna and Zotor, 2008; Aral, Holmes, Padian, and Cates, 1996; Arbabi, Nezami, Hooshyar, and Delavari, 2018). Without the intervention of winds or drafts, the distance over which airborne infection can take place is short, say 10 to 20 feet (Acemoglu and Johnson, 2007; Adda, 2016; Alloul, Sauriol, Kennedy, Laurier, Tessier, Novosel, and Contandriopoulos, 1998). This mode of transmission occurs in COVID-19 disease responsible for the 2019–2020 pandemic. In contrast, arthropod transmission takes place by an insect, either mechanically through contaminated proboscis or contaminated feet. It can also be transmitted biologically when there is growth or replication of an organism in the arthropod (Abegunde and Stanciole, 2008; Abramowitz, Lacau Saint Guily, Moyal-Barracco, Bergeron, Borne, Dahlab, and Bénard, 2018). Biological transmission involves certain biological processes such as passing a stage of development of the infecting agent in an intermediate host (Ozmen, Kurşun, and Ozcelik, 2005; Paarlberg, Hillberg, Lee, and Mathews, 2008; Paisley, Vraa-Andersen, Dybkjaer, Møller, Christensen, Mousing, and Agger, 1993). It is the opposite of mechanical transmission. In contact transmission the disease agent is transferred directly by biting, sucking, chewing or indirectly by inhalation of droplets, drinking of contaminated water, or by traveling in contaminated vehicles (Bonds, Keenan, Rohani, and Sachs, 2010; Boni, Galvani, Wickelgren, and Malani, 2013; Bonovas and Nikolopoulos, 2012).

Cyclopropagative transmission occurs when the agent undergoes both development and multiplication in the transmitting vehicle (Espinoza, Terashima, Herrera-Velit, and Marcos, 2010; Ezzati, Vander Hoorn, Lawes, Leach, James, Lopez, and Murray, 2005). In developmental transmission the agent undergoes some development in the transmission vehicle (Buckley, 1984; Budke, Jiamin, Qian, and Torgerson, 2005; Bundy, Arámbulo III, and Grey, 1983; Buzby and Roberts, 2009). Fecal-oral transmission occurs when the infectious agent is shed by the infected host in feces and acquired by the susceptible host through ingestion of contaminated material (Bwire, Munier, Ouedraogo, Heyerdahl, Komakech, Kagirita, and Makumbi, 2017; Canali, Aragrande, Angheben, Capelli, Drigo, Gobbi, and Cassini, 2020). Horizontal transmission occurs when there is lateral spread to others in the same group and at the same time or a spread to contemporaries (Yi-Xin and Manderson, 2005; Zadoks, 2008; Zhan, Li, Wang, Sun, Geng, Xiong, and de Hoog, 2015; Zhang, Song, Cai, and Zhou, 2008). Propagative transmission occurs when the agent multiplies in the transmission vehicle (Pal, Kerorsa, Marami, and Kandi, 2020; Paterson, Otte, Slingenbergh, Wint, and Rogers,

2000; Pearce and Merletti, 2006). Vertical transmission occurs from one generation to the next (Jenkins, Baingana, Ahmad, McDaid, and Atun, 2011; Johnson, Alvarez-Pasquin, Bijl, Franco, Gaillat, Clara, and Weinke, 2015). For instance, this can be transovarially or by intrauterine infection of the fetus (Abegunde and Stanciole, 2008; Abramowitz, Lacau Saint Guily, Moyal-Barracco, Bergeron, Borne, Dahlab, and Bénard, 2018). There are also retroviruses that are transmitted in the germline, in which case their genetic material is integrated into the DNA of either the ovum or sperm (Kim and Goldie, 2008; Klein, Laxminarayan, Smith, and Gilligan, 2007; Klepac, Laxminarayan, and Grenfell, 2011).

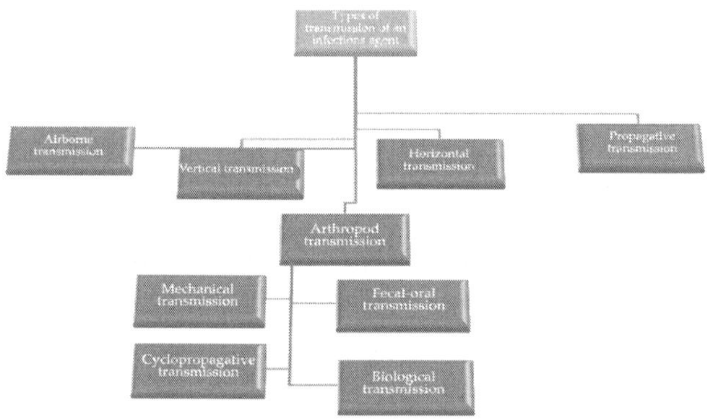

Preparations for an epidemic include having a disease surveillance system (Chen, Li, Hsieh, Chang, Lee, Lee, and Ko, 2012; Conover, Pitt, Kessler, DuBow, and Sanborn, 1995; Crump, Murdoch, and Baker, 2001). They also refer to the ability to quickly dispatch emergency workers, especially local-based emergency workers (Weycker, Edelsberg, Oster, and Tino, 2005; Wu, Perrings, Kinzig, Collins, Minteer, and Daszak, 2017; Yach, Stuckler, and Brownell, 2006). In doing so, that authorities identify a legitimate way to guarantee the safety and health of health workers (Perry and Randolph, 1999; Philipson, 2000; Philipson and Posner, 1996; Pongchaiyakul, Songpattanasilp, and Taechakraichana, 2008). Effective preparations for a response to a pandemic are multi-layered (Uusküla, Müürsepp, Kawai, Raag, Jürisson, and Pillsbury, 2013; Vanni, Karnon, Madan, White, Edmunds, Foss, and Legood, 2011). The first layer is a disease surveillance system (St George, 1986; Steben and Duarte-Franco, 2007; Stehr-Green and Schantz, 1987; Stuckler, 2008; Stuckler and Siegel, 2011). Tanzania, for example, runs a national lab that runs testing for 200 health sites and tracks the spread of infectious diseases. The next layer is the actual response to an emergency (Acemoglu and Johnson, 2007; Adda, 2016; Alloul, Sauriol, Kennedy, Laurier, Tessier, Novosel, and Contandriopoulos, 1998). According to U.S.-based columnist Michael Gerson in 2015, only the U.S. military and NATO have the global capability to respond to such an emergency (Amuna and Zotor, 2008; Aral, Holmes, Padian, and Cates, 1996; Arbabi, Nezami, Hooshyar, and Delavari, 2018). Despite the most extensive preparatory measures, a fast-spreading pandemic may easily exceed and overwhelm existing healthcare resources (Krieger, 2001a, b; Lemma, 1969; Liu, Maniadakis, Gray, and Rayner, 2002; López, Torné, Franco, San-Martin, Viayna, Barrull, and Perulero, 2018). Consequently, by taking early and aggressive mitigating action the "epidemic Curve Flattening" can be achieved (Armelagos, Brown, and Turner, 2005; Arokiasamy and Krishnan, 1994; Arora, 2001, 2005; Arredondo and Zúñiga, 2004). Such measures usually consist on non-pharmacological interventions such as social or physical distancing, aggressive contact tracing, "stay-at-home" orders (Suhrcke, Stuckler, Suk, Desai, Senek, McKee, and Rechel, 2011; Šumilo, Bormane, Asokliene, Vasilenko, Golovljova, Avsic-Zupanc, and Randolph, 2008). It may also include the deliberate use of appropriate personal protective equipment including masks, gloves, and other physical barriers to spread (Poundstone, Strathdee, and Celentano, 2004; Pritchett, Thilmany, and Johnson, 2005; Pugliatti, Beghi, Forsgren, Ekman, and Sobocki, 2007). In the next section, we examine the spatial scope of epidemics.

1.2. EPIDEMICS AND THEIR SPATIAL SCOPE

Improvements in our understanding of the spatial-temporal variation with regards to the spread of infectious diseases is a necessary step when contemplating the development of innovative strategies (Bergevoet, Van Schaik, Veling, Backus, and Franken, 2009; Binder, 1988; Bolos, Bacarea, and Marusteri, 2011). Such innovative strategies could help to ameliorate the impact of disease epidemicsDisease epidemics on morbidity and mortality rates across the globe (Arredondo and Zúñiga, 2006; Backer, van Roermund, Fischer, van Asseldonk, and Bergevoet, 2015; Bartsch, Hotez, Hertenstein, Diemert, Zapf, Bottazzi, and Lee, 2016). Quantitative approaches that rely on mathematical models and methodology from the field of spatial epidemiology are being increasingly used to address questions relating to the geographic distribution of infectious diseases and the design of control strategies (Howe, Häsler, and Stärk, 2013; Howe et al., 2012). As a result of which researchers have started studying the spatial epidemiology of conditions such as influenza, cholera, malaria, tuberculosis, HIV, measles, Zika virus, and Ebola virus disease (Raut, 2004; Rehm, Mathers, Popova, Thavorncharoensap, Teerawattananon, and Patra, 2009; Rich and Perry, 2011). Given the sharp economic decline that can arise out of disease epidemics (see Figure 1.2 for an example of the economic devastation on the US economy following the COVID-19 epidemic); such planning is necessary.

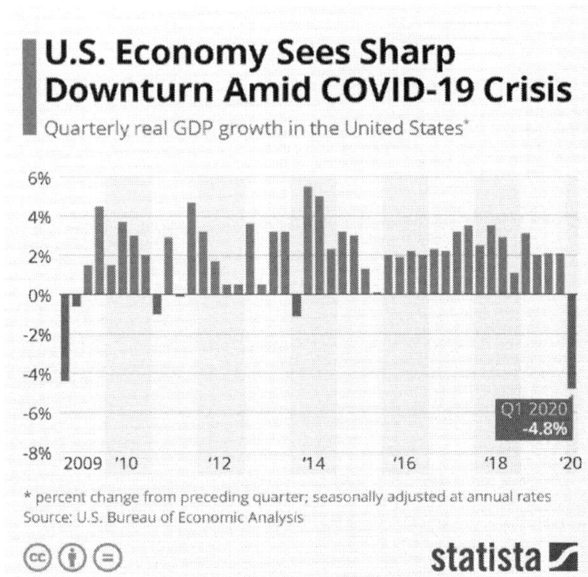

Figure 1.2. USA economy shrinks during COVID-19 crisis.

Source: Statista via the World Economic Forum.

There are many considerations in the process of mapping spatial epidemiology (Hart and Halden, 2020; Häsler, Howe, and Stärk, 2011; Henschke, Kamper, and Maher, 2015; Hochberg, 1992). First, it may involve explaining the spatial patterns of infectious diseases through quantitative analyzes that make use of spatially resolved socio-demographic and epidemiological datasets (Markos and Abdela, 2016; Martin and Shepherd, 2009; McGuinness, McGlynn, Johnson, MacIntyre, Batty, Burns, and McGinty, 2012). The spacio-temporal transmission dynamics of any disease epidemic can be predicted with greater accuracy as a result of these activities as they increase our understanding of these activities (Foxman, 2002; Garner, Whan, Gard, and Phillips, 2001; Gayle and Hill,

2001; Gottstein, Pozio, and Nöckler, 2009). This may help when predicting the impact of control interventions that are driven by geographical factors (Moné, Ibikounlé, Massougbodji, and Mouahid, 2010; Morand, 2004; Moro, Budke, Schantz, Vasquez, Santivanez, and Villavicencio, 2011). Ultimately, the authorities may use the information that is garnered when designing or evaluating optimal resource allocation strategies that incorporate a spatial component in the management of the outbreak (Eaton and Groopman, 2013; Eckelman, Sherman, and MacNeill, 2018; Egger, 2011; Elbe, 2007; Ernst and Hay, 1994). It is anticipated that such a detailed information-gathering process will help in generating cost-effectiveness analyzes that incorporate a spatial component (Oleś, Gudowska-Nowak, and Kleczkowski, 2012; Otte, Nugent, and McLeod, 2004; Ozawa, Portnoy, Getaneh, Clark, Knoll, Bishai, and Patwardhan, 2016). Finally, the investigations may involve analyzing inequities in healthcare based on geography, which are currently key components of the impact of these epidemics (Rogers, Carolin, Vaught, and Compton, 2011; Ronohardjo and Rastiko, 1982; Sachs, 2001; Sachs and Malaney, 2002).

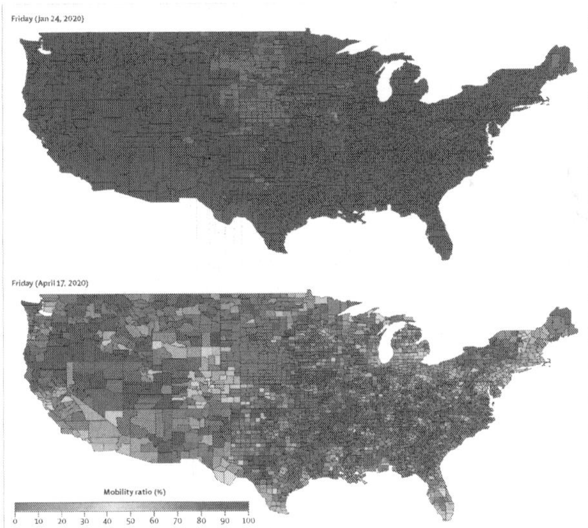

Source: https://www.thelancet.com/journals/laninf/article/PIIS1473-3099(20)30553-3/fulltext

Spatial epidemiology is a subfield of epidemiology focused on the study of the spatial distribution of health outcomes. It is closely related to health geography (Bausch and Schwarz, 2014; Bausch et al., 2001; Benner,

Carabin, Sánchez-Serrano, Budke, and Carmena, 2010). Specifically, spatial epidemiology is concerned with the description and examination of disease and its geographic variations (Purevdawa, Moon, Baigalmaa, Davaajav, Smith, and Vermund, 1997; Ramesh, Malla, Raju, Sehgal, Ganguly, Mahajan, and Dilawari, 1990). This is done in consideration of demographic, environmental, behavioral, socioeconomic, genetic, and the risk factors of infections (Borghol, Suderman, McArdle, Racine, Hallett, Pembrey, and Szyf, 2012; Brandes, 2008; Brown, Lipscomb, and Snyder, 2001). There are many different types of studies that are undertaken as part of the process of understanding spatial epidemiology (Tapia, 2003; Torgerson and Dowling, 2001; Torgerson, Carmona, and Bonifacino, 2000; Uddin Khan, Atanasova, Krueger, Ramirez, and Gray, 2013). A case in point is the use of disease mapping. Disease maps are visual representations of intricate geographic data that provide a quick overview of said information (Saleha, 1991; Sibert, Rigaud, Delavierre, and Labat, 2010; Skrepnek and Skrepnek, 2004; Sloane, 2009; Sockett, 1993). In order to aid policy making and allocation of resources, disease maps can be used as a medium of explanation (Peckham, 2013; Perrings et al., 2002, 2014).

Geographic correlation studies attempt to study the geographical factors and their effects on geographically differentiated health outcomes (Daily, and Ehrlich, 1996; Deogaonkar, Hutubessy, Van Der Putten, Evers, and Jit, 2012; Dorn, 1992; Ducrotoy, Bertu, Ocholi, Gusi, Bryssinckx, Welburn, and Moriyon, 2014). Measured on an ecologic scale; these factors include environmental variables (quality of surrounding space), socioeconomic, and demographic statistics (income and race), or even lifestyle choices (nutrition or diet) of the population groups under study (Fenichel, 2013; Fenichel et al., 2011; Fogel, 1994). This approach has the convenience of being able to employ the already available data from various surveying sources (Narrod, Zinsstag, and Tiongco, 2012; Nascimento and de Oliveira, 2014; O'Brien, Lahue, Caro, and Davidson, 2007). Others may hope to make use of clustering, disease clusters, and surveillance (Casamassimo, Thikkurissy, Edelstein, and Maiorini, 2009; Castro, Wilson, and Bloom, 2017). Disease clusters, or spatial groupings based on proximity and characteristically related epidemics (Abegunde and Stanciole, 2008; Abramowitz, Lacau Saint Guily, Moyal-Barracco, Bergeron, Borne, Dahlab, and Bénard, 2018). While the term itself is relatively poorly defined, it generally implies an excess of cases above some background rate bounded in time and space (Acemoglu and Johnson, 2007; Adda, 2016; Alloul, Sauriol, Kennedy, Laurier, Tessier, Novosel, and Contandriopoulos, 1998). Although clustering is not the most precise method for spatial analysis, it can and has proved useful for health-related surveillance and monitoring (Amuna and Zotor, 2008; Aral, Holmes, Padian, and Cates, 1996; Arbabi, Nezami, Hooshyar, and Delavari, 2018).

Owing to the complexity of the statistical models that are deployed to draw up this research, the data analysis and the interpretation of results should be carried out by qualified statisticians (Armelagos, Brown, and Turner, 2005; Arokiasamy and Krishnan, 1994; Arora, 2001, 2005; Arredondo and Zúñiga, 2004). Sometimes, the proliferation of errors in disease mapping has led to inefficient decision-making, implementation of inappropriate health policies and negative impact on the advancement of scientific knowledge (Arredondo and Zúñiga, 2006; Backer, van Roermund, Fischer, van Asseldonk, and Bergevoet, 2015; Bartsch, Hotez, Hertenstein, Diemert, Zapf, Bottazzi, and Lee, 2016). Therefore, many challenges arise before, during, and after spatial epidemiology mapping (Bausch and Schwarz, 2014; Bausch et al., 2001; Benner, Carabin, Sánchez-Serrano, Budke, and Carmena, 2010). One of those challenges is the difficulty of accessing good quality data (Bergevoet, Van Schaik, Veling, Backus, and Franken, 2009; Binder, 1988; Bolos, Bacarea, and Marusteri, 2011). Since spatial epidemiology is almost entirely based on the analysis of data and its various visual representations, it is imperative that data collection methods be routine, accurate, and publicly available (Bonds, Keenan, Rohani, and Sachs, 2010; Boni, Galvani, Wickelgren, and Malani, 2013; Bonovas and Nikolopoulos, 2012). With the advent of specialized and accurate health equipment and global information networks, these methods can be relatively and easily improved (Borghol, Suderman, McArdle, Racine, Hallett, Pembrey, and Szyf, 2012; Brandes, 2008; Brown, Lipscomb, and Snyder, 2001). Given the right tools and processes, compiling and standardizing data can also be done efficiently and usefully (Buckley, 1984; Budke, Jiamin, Qian, and Torgerson, 2005; Bundy, Arámbulo III, and Grey, 1983; Buzby and Roberts, 2009).

There are enhanced requirements for data protection and confidentiality when the specific epidemic carries stigma, such as was the case with HIV/AIDS, tuberculosis, the plagues, and leprosy (Bwire, Munier, Ouedraogo, Heyerdahl, Komakech, Kagirita, and Makumbi, 2017; Canali, Aragrande, Angheben, Capelli, Drigo, Gobbi, and Cassini, 2020). At the present moment, legislation in the United States regarding individual human rights are gaining increasing support, especially in regards to the confidentiality of personal health data and consent over its use in medical investigations (Casamassimo, Thikkurissy, Edelstein, and Maiorini, 2009; Castro, Wilson, and Bloom, 2017). Safe and secure data is a crucial aspect of successful epidemiologic research (Chen, Li, Hsieh, Chang, Lee, Lee, and Ko, 2012; Conover, Pitt, Kessler, DuBow, and Sanborn, 1995; Crump, Murdoch, and Baker, 2001). Not only does it increase confidence in the system, but it also increases the possibility of communities getting involved (Daily, and Ehrlich, 1996; Deogaonkar, Hutubessy, Van Der Putten, Evers, and Jit, 2012; Dorn, 1992; Ducrotoy, Bertu, Ocholi, Gusi, Bryssinckx, Welburn, and Moriyon, 2014).

There is a risk of exposure assessment and mapping in practical and analytical terms (Eaton and Groopman, 2013; Eckelman, Sherman, and MacNeill, 2018; Egger, 2011; Elbe, 2007; Ernst and Hay, 1994). Because it is always seen as an analytical weakness, the quality of exposure data, or reported accuracy of the spatial reach of epidemics, is especially important in spatial epidemiology (Espinoza, Terashima, Herrera-Velit, and Marcos, 2010; Ezzati, Vander Hoorn, Lawes, Leach, James, Lopez, and Murray, 2005). With the more mainstream use of geographic information systems, the capabilities of spatial interpolation and mapping have been significantly improved (Fenichel, 2013; Fenichel et al., 2011; Fogel, 1994). Yet, these still greatly depend on the precision and legitimacy of the source data commissioned. Researchers are particularly interested in geostatistical analyzes of data, and transmission or economic models (Foxman, 2002; Garner, Whan, Gard, and Phillips, 2001; Gayle and Hill, 2001; Gottstein, Pozio, and Nöckler, 2009).

There have been many important ecological and public health questions related to the transmission of infectious disease that neither need, nor would benefit from, a mechanistic model in which space is represented explicitly (Hart and Halden, 2020; Häsler, Howe, and Stärk, 2011; Henschke, Kamper, and Maher, 2015; Hochberg, 1992). In many instances, the concept of the average behavior of a large population is sufficient to provide genuinely useful insight and to extract good information from the data that are available (Howe, Häsler, and Stärk, 2013; Howe et al., 2012). However, the importance of the spatial component of many transmission systems is being increasingly recognized (Jenkins, Baingana, Ahmad, McDaid, and Atun, 2011; Johnson, Alvarez-Pasquin, Bijl, Franco, Gaillat, Clara, and Weinke, 2015). While there is a need to consider spatially heterogeneous interventions, it is clearly essential to represent the location of hosts and the pattern of transmission (Kim and Goldie, 2008; Klein, Laxminarayan, Smith, and Gilligan, 2007; Klepac, Laxminarayan, and Grenfell, 2011). Sometimes the location of the hosts in space is clearly defined and easily measured, e.g., with regards to plant systems and some livestock systems (Krieger, 2001a, b; Lemma, 1969; Liu, Maniadakis, Gray, and Rayner, 2002; López, Torné, Franco, San-Martin, Viayna, Barrull, and Perulero, 2018). However, in the case of humans and wild animals; the single location assigned to a host can at best represent the average deduced from the complex social behavior of each individual (Markos and Abdela, 2016; Martin and Shepherd, 2009; McGuinness, McGlynn, Johnson, MacIntyre, Batty, Burns, and McGinty, 2012).

If it is thought that the aggregate characteristics of epidemic incidence are being driven by spatial aspects of transmission (e.g., waves), it is difficult to investigate data from these systems with models that do not represent space in some way (Moné, Ibikounlé, Massougbodji, and Mouahid, 2010; Morand, 2004; Moro, Budke, Schantz, Vasquez, Santivanez, and Villavicencio, 2011). Where data sets are provided with high spatial resolution, even when the primary hypotheses of interest for a given phenomenon does not relate directly to spatial effects, it is often necessary to account for spatial processes in order to discount plausible alternate explanations for an observed feature in the data (Narrod, Zinsstag, and Tiongco, 2012; Nascimento and de Oliveira, 2014; O'Brien, Lahue, Caro, and Davidson, 2007). In the next section, we consider the timelines of disease epidemics.

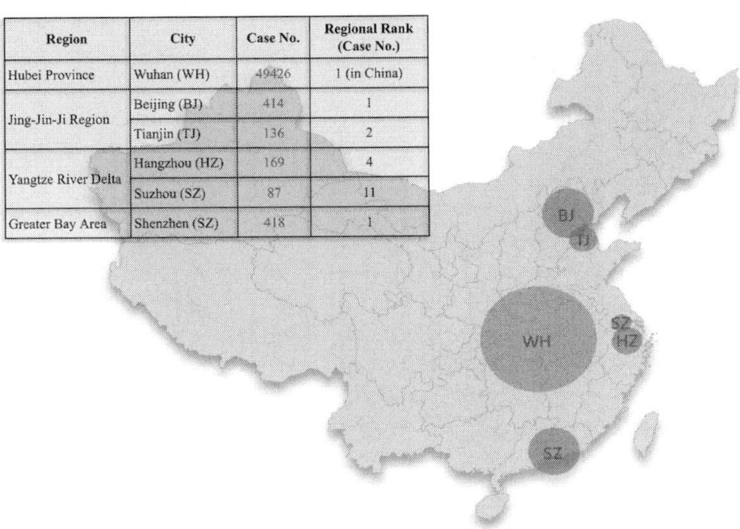

Region	City	Case No.	Regional Rank (Case No.)
Hubei Province	Wuhan (WH)	49426	1 (in China)
Jing-Jin-Ji Region	Beijing (BJ)	414	1
	Tianjin (TJ)	136	2
Yangtze River Delta	Hangzhou (HZ)	169	4
	Suzhou (SZ)	87	11
Greater Bay Area	Shenzhen (SZ)	418	1

Source: Eclinical medicine, a Lancet publication. https://www.thelancet.com/journals/eclinm/article/PIIS2589-5370(20)30098-5/fulltext

The geographical locations and the disease situations (total number of cases from Dec. 2019 to Feb. 2020) of six major cities selected in this study: Wuhan, Beijing, Tianjin, Hangzhou, Suzhou, and Shenzhen.

1.3. THE TIMELINES OF DISEASE EPIDEMICS

The timelines of disease epidemicsDisease epidemics are an important consideration when planning a response, as well as any other appropriate preventative measures (Oleś, Gudowska-Nowak, and Kleczkowski, 2012; Otte, Nugent, and McLeod, 2004; Ozawa, Portnoy, Getaneh, Clark, Knoll, Bishai, and Patwardhan, 2016). Throughout history, the major epidemics have been more or less identified by their timeline (Ozmen, Kurşun, and Ozcelik, 2005; Paarlberg, Hillberg, Lee, and Mathews, 2008; Paisley, Vraa-Andersen, Dybkjaer, Møller, Christensen, Mousing, and Agger, 1993). Currently, the world is in the midst of 2020; COVID-19 pandemic, although the exact timelines have not yet been fully established. Where there are predictions of a quick recovery and return to normal, these have often been disappointed by the reality. One of the things that all these pandemics share (regardless of their timeline), is the significant impact that they have on the global economy (Pal, Kerorsa, Marami, and Kandi, 2020; Paterson, Otte, Slingenbergh, Wint, and Rogers, 2000; Pearce and Merletti, 2006). In Figure 1.3, we see the impact of the Influenza epidemic on the global economy.

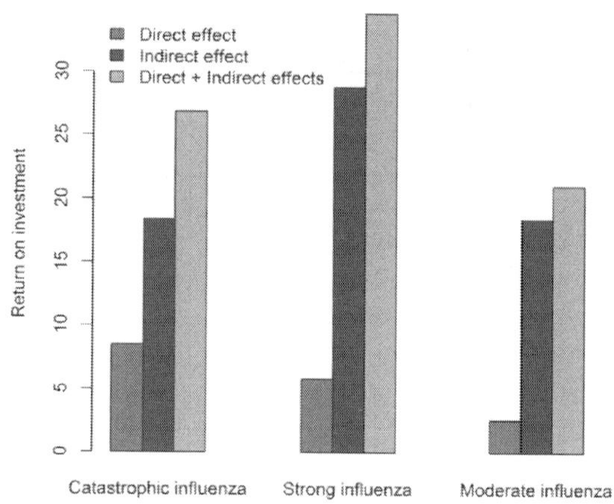

Figure 1.3. Impact of different influenza levels on the economy.

Source: PLoS.

Existing literature has recorded a number of pandemics and their respective timelines for posterity and also to reflect in terms of the response from the global economies (Peckham, 2013; Perrings et al., 2002, 2014). A pandemic is an epidemic of an infectious disease that has spread across a large region (Perry and Randolph, 1999; Philipson, 2000; Philipson and Posner, 1996; Pongchaiyakul, Songpattanasilp, and Taechakraichana, 2008). A pandemic may involve several continents or even span the entire world (Poundstone, Strathdee, and Celentano, 2004; Pritchett, Thilmany, and Johnson, 2005; Pugliatti, Beghi, Forsgren, Ekman, and Sobocki, 2007). A widespread endemic disease with a stable number of infected people is not a pandemic (Purevdawa, Moon, Baigalmaa, Davaajav, Smith, and Vermund, 1997; Ramesh, Malla, Raju, Sehgal, Ganguly, Mahajan, and Dilawari, 1990). Widespread endemic diseases with a stable number of infected people such as recurrences of seasonal influenza are generally excluded as they occur simultaneously in large regions of the globe rather than being spread worldwide (Raut, 2004; Rehm, Mathers, Popova, Thavorncharoensap, Teerawattananon, and Patra, 2009; Rich and Perry, 2011). Throughout human history, there have been a number of pandemics of diseases such as smallpox and tuberculosis (Rogers, Carolin, Vaught, and Compton, 2011; Ronohardjo and Rastiko, 1982; Sachs, 2001; Sachs and Malaney, 2002). The most fatal pandemic in recorded history was the Black Death (also known as The Plague), which killed an estimated 75–200 million people in the 14th century (Saleha, 1991; Sibert, Rigaud, Delavierre, and Labat, 2010; Skrepnek and Skrepnek, 2004; Sloane, 2009; Sockett, 1993). The term was not used yet but was for later pandemics, including the 1918 influenza pandemic or the Spanish flu (St George, 1986; Steben and Duarte-Franco, 2007; Stehr-Green and Schantz, 1987; Stuckler, 2008; Stuckler and Siegel, 2011). Current pandemics include COVID-19 and HIV/AIDS (Suhrcke, Stuckler, Suk, Desai, Senek, McKee, and Rechel, 2011; Šumilo, Bormane, Asokliene, Vasilenko, Golovljova, Avsic-Zupanc, and Randolph, 2008).

A pandemic is an epidemic occurring on a scale that crosses international boundaries, usually affecting people at a worldwide level (Tapia, 2003; Torgerson and Dowling, 2001; Torgerson, Carmona, and Bonifacino, 2000; Uddin Khan, Atanasova, Krueger, Ramirez, and Gray, 2013). A disease or condition is not a pandemic merely because it is widespread or kills many people; it must also be infectious (Uusküla, Müürsepp, Kawai, Raag, Jürisson, and Pillsbury, 2013; Vanni, Karnon, Madan, White, Edmunds, Foss, and Legood, 2011). For instance, cancer is responsible for many deaths but is not considered a pandemic because the disease is neither infectious nor contagious (Weycker, Edelsberg, Oster, and Tino, 2005; Wu, Perrings, Kinzig, Collins, Minteer, and Daszak, 2017; Yach, Stuckler, and Brownell, 2006). The WHO previously applied a six-stage classification to describe the process by which a novel influenza virus moves from the first few infections in humans through to a pandemic (Yi-Xin and Manderson, 2005; Zadoks, 2008; Zhan, Li, Wang, Sun, Geng, Xiong, and de Hoog, 2015; Zhang, Song, Cai, and Zhou, 2008). It starts when mostly animals are infected with a virus and a few cases where animals infect people (Narrod, Zinsstag, and Tiongco, 2012; Nascimento and de Oliveira, 2014; O'Brien, Lahue, Caro, and Davidson, 2007). The disease then escalates to a stage where there is transmission directly between people (Fenichel, 2013; Fenichel et al., 2011; Fogel, 1994). The final stage of the pattern is when the viral infections in humans is spread worldwide (Casamassimo, Thikkurissy, Edelstein, and Maiorini, 2009; Castro, Wilson, and Bloom, 2017). In February 2020, a WHO spokesperson clarified that there is no official category for a pandemic.

In planning for a possible influenza pandemic, the WHO published a document on pandemic preparedness guidance in 1999, revised in 2005 and 2009, defining phases and appropriate actions for each phase in an aide-mémoire titled WHO Pandemic Phase Descriptions and Main Actions by Phase (Daily, and Ehrlich, 1996; Deogaonkar, Hutubessy, Van Der Putten, Evers, and Jit, 2012; Dorn, 1992; Ducrotoy, Bertu, Ocholi, Gusi, Bryssinckx, Welburn, and Moriyon, 2014). The 2009 revision, was finalized in February 2009 and included the definition of pandemic and elaborated the phases that would lead to the declaration of pandemic. In 2009, H1N1 virus pandemic was neither on the horizon at that time nor mentioned in the document (Peckham, 2013; Perrings et al., 2002, 2014). All versions of this document refer to influenza (Saleha, 1991; Sibert, Rigaud, Delavierre, and Labat, 2010; Skrepnek and Skrepnek, 2004; Sloane, 2009; Sockett, 1993). The phases are defined by the spread of the disease; virulence and mortality are not mentioned in the current WHO definition, although these factors had previously been added (Tapia, 2003; Torgerson and Dowling, 2001; Torgerson, Carmona, and Bonifacino, 2000; Uddin Khan, Atanasova, Krueger, Ramirez, and Gray, 2013). In 2014, The United States CDC introduced an analogous framework to the WHO's pandemic stages titled the Pandemic Intervals Framework (Borghol, Suderman, McArdle, Racine, Hallett, Pembrey, and Szyf, 2012; Brandes, 2008; Brown, Lipscomb, and Snyder, 2001). It includes two pre-pandemic intervals including investigation and recognition (Purevdawa, Moon, Baigalmaa, Davaajav, Smith, and Vermund, 1997; Ramesh, Malla, Raju, Sehgal, Ganguly,

Mahajan, and Dilawari, 1990). There are four pandemic intervals including: initiation, acceleration, deceleration, and preparation (Bausch and Schwarz, 2014; Bausch et al., 2001; Benner, Carabin, Sánchez-Serrano, Budke, and Carmena, 2010). The staged classification also includes a table defining the intervals and mapping them to the WHO pandemic stages (Rogers, Carolin, Vaught, and Compton, 2011; Ronohardjo and Rastiko, 1982; Sachs, 2001; Sachs and Malaney, 2002).

In human history, it is generally zoonoses such as influenza and tuberculosis which have been responsible for most of the widespread outbreaks, occurring as a result of the domestication of animals (Oleś, Gudowska-Nowak, and Kleczkowski, 2012; Otte, Nugent, and McLeod, 2004; Ozawa, Portnoy, Getaneh, Clark, Knoll, Bishai, and Patwardhan, 2016). There have been a number of particularly significant epidemics that deserve mention above the "mere" destruction of cities:

- **Plague of Athens (430 to 426 BC):** During the Peloponnesian War, typhoid fever killed a quarter of the Athenian troops and a quarter of the population (Eaton and Groopman, 2013; Eckelman, Sherman, and MacNeill, 2018; Egger, 2011; Elbe, 2007; Ernst and Hay, 1994). This disease fatally weakened the dominance of Athens, but the sheer virulence of the disease prevented its wider spread., i.e., it killed off its hosts at a rate faster than the rate of spread (Moné, Ibikounlé, Massougbodji, and Mouahid, 2010; Morand, 2004; Moro, Budke, Schantz, Vasquez, Santivanez, and Villavicencio, 2011). The exact cause of the plague was unknown for many years (Foxman, 2002; Garner, Whan, Gard, and Phillips, 2001; Gayle and Hill, 2001; Gottstein, Pozio, and Nöckler, 2009). In January 2006, researchers from the University of Athens analyzed teeth recovered from a mass grave underneath the city and confirmed the presence of bacteria responsible for typhoid (Markos and Abdela, 2016; Martin and Shepherd, 2009; McGuinness, McGlynn, Johnson, MacIntyre, Batty, Burns, and McGinty, 2012).
- **Antonine Plague (165 to 180 AD):** Possibly measles or smallpox brought to the Italian peninsula by soldiers returning from the Near East (Hart and Halden, 2020; Häsler, Howe, and Stärk, 2011; Henschke, Kamper, and Maher, 2015; Hochberg, 1992). This epidemic killed a quarter of those infected, up to 5 million in total (Raut, 2004; Rehm, Mathers, Popova, Thavorncharoensap, Teerawattananon, and Patra, 2009; Rich and Perry, 2011).

- **Plague of Cyprian (251–266 AD):** A second outbreak of what may have been the same disease as the Antonine Plague, which allegedly killed about 5,000 people a day in Rome (Howe, Häsler, and Stärk, 2013; Howe et al., 2012).
- **Plague of Justinian (541 to 750 AD):** The first recorded outbreak of the bubonic plague started in Egypt and reached Constantinople the following spring, killing 10,000 a day at its height, and perhaps 40% of the city's inhabitants (Arredondo and Zúñiga, 2006; Backer, van Roermund, Fischer, van Asseldonk, and Bergevoet, 2015; Bartsch, Hotez, Hertenstein, Diemert, Zapf, Bottazzi, and Lee, 2016). The plague went on to eliminate a quarter to half the human population of the known world (Bergevoet, Van Schaik, Veling, Backus, and Franken, 2009; Binder, 1988; Bolos, Bacarea, and Marusteri, 2011). It caused Europe's population to drop by around 50% between 550 AD and 700 AD (Suhrcke, Stuckler, Suk, Desai, Senek, McKee, and Rechel, 2011; Šumilo, Bormane, Asokliene, Vasilenko, Golovljova, Avsic-Zupanc, and Randolph, 2008).
- **Black Death (1331 to 1353):** The total number of deaths worldwide is estimated at 75 to 200 million for the Black Death (Poundstone, Strathdee, and Celentano, 2004; Pritchett, Thilmany, and Johnson, 2005; Pugliatti, Beghi, Forsgren, Ekman, and Sobocki, 2007). About 800 years after the last outbreak, the plague returned to Europe (Armelagos, Brown, and Turner, 2005; Arokiasamy and Krishnan, 1994; Arora, 2001, 2005; Arredondo and Zúñiga, 2004). Starting in Asia, the disease reached the Mediterranean and western Europe in 1348 (possibly from Italian merchants fleeing fighting in Crimea), and killed an estimated 20 to 30 million Europeans in 6 years (Krieger, 2001a, b; Lemma, 1969; Liu, Maniadakis, Gray, and Rayner, 2002; López, Torné, Franco, San-Martin, Viayna, Barrull, and Perulero, 2018). This represented a third of the total population and up to a half in the worst-affected urban areas (Amuna and Zotor, 2008; Aral, Holmes, Padian, and Cates, 1996; Arbabi, Nezami, Hooshyar, and Delavari, 2018). It was the first of a cycle of European plague epidemics that continued until the 18th century (Acemoglu and Johnson, 2007; Adda, 2016; Alloul, Sauriol, Kennedy, Laurier, Tessier, Novosel, and Contandriopoulos, 1998). There were more than 100 plague epidemics in Europe during this period (St

George, 1986; Steben and Duarte-Franco, 2007; Stehr-Green and Schantz, 1987; Stuckler, 2008; Stuckler and Siegel, 2011). The disease recurred in England every 2 to 5 years from 1361 to 1480 (Uusküla, Müürsepp, Kawai, Raag, Jürisson, and Pillsbury, 2013; Vanni, Karnon, Madan, White, Edmunds, Foss, and Legood, 2011). By the 1370s, England's population was reduced by 50% (Perry and Randolph, 1999; Philipson, 2000; Philipson and Posner, 1996; Pongchaiyakul, Songpattanasilp, and Taechakraichana, 2008). The Great Plague of London of 1665–1666 was the last major outbreak of the plague in England and killed approximately 100,000 people or about 20% of London's population (Weycker, Edelsberg, Oster, and Tino, 2005; Wu, Perrings, Kinzig, Collins, Minteer, and Daszak, 2017; Yach, Stuckler, and Brownell, 2006).

- **Third Plague Pandemic (1855):** Starting in China, it spread into India, where 10 million people died (Chen, Li, Hsieh, Chang, Lee, Lee, and Ko, 2012; Conover, Pitt, Kessler, DuBow, and Sanborn, 1995; Crump, Murdoch, and Baker, 2001). During this pandemic, the United States saw its first outbreak, which was known as the San Francisco plague of 1900–1904 (Kim and Goldie, 2008; Klein, Laxminarayan, Smith, and Gilligan, 2007; Klepac, Laxminarayan, and Grenfell, 2011). Today, sporadic cases of plague still occur in the western United States (Abegunde and Stanciole, 2008; Abramowitz, Lacau Saint Guily, Moyal-Barracco, Bergeron, Borne, Dahlab, and Bénard, 2018).
- **The 1918 Flu Pandemic:** This infected half a billion people around the world, including on remote Pacific islands and in the Arctic, killing between 20 and 100 million (Jenkins, Baingana, Ahmad, McDaid, and Atun, 2011; Johnson, Alvarez-Pasquin, Bijl, Franco, Gaillat, Clara, and Weinke, 2015). Most influenza outbreaks disproportionately kill the very young or the very old, with higher survival rates for those in between (Pal, Kerorsa, Marami, and Kandi, 2020; Paterson, Otte, Slingenbergh, Wint, and Rogers, 2000; Pearce and Merletti, 2006). However, the 1918 pandemic had an unusually high mortality rate for young adults (Yi-Xin and Manderson, 2005; Zadoks, 2008; Zhan, Li, Wang, Sun, Geng, Xiong, and de Hoog, 2015; Zhang, Song, Cai, and Zhou, 2008). It killed more people in 25 weeks than AIDS did in its first 25 years (Bwire, Munier, Ouedraogo, Heyerdahl, Komakech, Kagirita, and Makumbi, 2017; Canali, Aragrande,

Angheben, Capelli, Drigo, Gobbi, and Cassini, 2020). Mass troop movements and close quarters during World War I caused it to mutate and spread faster, and the susceptibility of soldiers to the flu may have been increased by stress, malnourishment, and chemical attacks (Buckley, 1984; Budke, Jiamin, Qian, and Torgerson, 2005; Bundy, Arámbulo III, and Grey, 1983; Buzby and Roberts, 2009). Improved transportation systems made it easier for soldiers, sailors, and civilian travelers to spread the disease (Espinoza, Terashima, Herrera-Velit, and Marcos, 2010; Ezzati, Vander Hoorn, Lawes, Leach, James, Lopez, and Murray, 2005).

The next section is about the people that are most affected by disease epidemicsDisease epidemics.

1.4. THE PEOPLE THAT ARE AFFECTED BY DISEASE EPIDEMICS

Typically, these disease outbreaks tended to severely impact on the urban poor (Eaton and Groopman, 2013; Eckelman, Sherman, and MacNeill, 2018; Egger, 2011; Elbe, 2007; Ernst and Hay, 1994). The same trend continues even today (Espinoza, Terashima, Herrera-Velit, and Marcos, 2010; Ezzati, Vander Hoorn, Lawes, Leach, James, Lopez, and Murray, 2005). After a steady decline in the number of countries suffering from epidemics in the period running from 1995 to 2010; there is a significant rise in the geographical spread of disease epidemicsDisease epidemics (see Figure 1.4). Some argue that this is due to the increase in travel and urbanization (Markos and Abdela, 2016; Martin and Shepherd, 2009; McGuinness, McGlynn, Johnson, MacIntyre, Batty, Burns, and McGinty, 2012). Where people are found in a state of economic distress, the disease epidemic is likely to make things much worse (Suhrcke, Stuckler, Suk, Desai, Senek, McKee, and Rechel, 2011; Šumilo, Bormane, Asokliene, Vasilenko, Golovljova, Avsic-Zupanc, and Randolph, 2008). That is why many of the public interventions tend to target the urban poor (Bergevoet, Van Schaik, Veling, Backus, and Franken, 2009; Binder, 1988; Bolos, Bacarea, and Marusteri, 2011). Such decisions will have been informed by experience of identifying poor urban populations as being particularly vulnerable to previous epidemics as we shall see in this séction (Tapia, 2003; Torgerson and Dowling, 2001; Torgerson, Carmona, and Bonifacino, 2000; Uddin Khan, Atanasova, Krueger, Ramirez, and Gray, 2013).

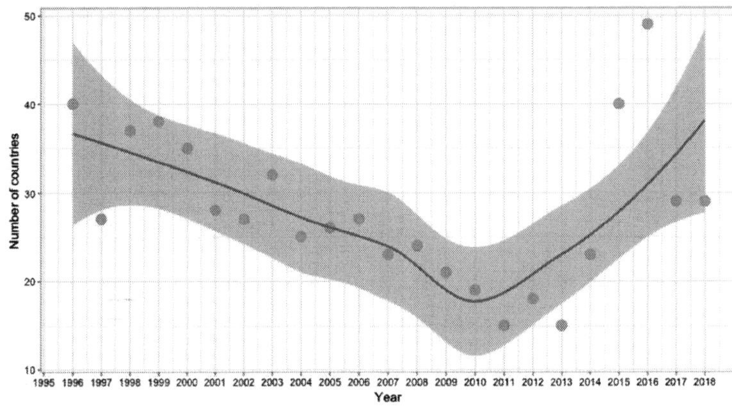

Figure 1.4. Number of countries facing disease outbreaks 1995–2018.

Source: World Economic Forum.

Encounters between European explorers and populations of the rest of the world often introduced epidemics of extraordinary virulence (Bonds, Keenan, Rohani, and Sachs, 2010; Boni, Galvani, Wickelgren, and Malani, 2013; Bonovas and Nikolopoulos, 2012). Disease killed part of the native population of the Canary Islands in the 16th century (Guanches). Half the native population of Hispaniola in 1518 was killed by smallpox (Ozmen, Kurşun, and Ozcelik, 2005; Paarlberg, Hillberg, Lee, and Mathews, 2008; Paisley, Vraa-Andersen, Dybkjaer, Møller, Christensen, Mousing, and Agger, 1993). Smallpox also ravaged Mexico in the 1520s, killing 150,000 in Tenochtitlan alone, including the emperor, and in Peru in the 1530s, proving beneficial to the European conquerors (Casamassimo, Thikkurissy, Edelstein, and Maiorini, 2009; Castro, Wilson, and Bloom, 2017). Measles killed a further 2 million Mexican natives in the 17th century (Poundstone, Strathdee, and Celentano, 2004; Pritchett, Thilmany, and Johnson, 2005; Pugliatti, Beghi, Forsgren, Ekman, and Sobocki, 2007). In 1618–1619, smallpox wiped out 90% of the Massachusetts Bay Native Americans (St George, 1986; Steben and Duarte-Franco, 2007; Stehr-Green and Schantz, 1987; Stuckler, 2008; Stuckler and Siegel, 2011). During the 1770s, smallpox killed at least 30% of the Pacific Northwest Native Americans. Smallpox epidemics in 1780–1782 and 1837–1838 brought devastation and drastic depopulation among the Plains Indians (Kim and Goldie, 2008; Klein, Laxminarayan, Smith, and Gilligan, 2007; Klepac, Laxminarayan, and Grenfell, 2011). Some believe the death of up to 95% of the Native American population of the New World was caused by Europeans introducing Old World diseases such as smallpox, measles, and influenza (Bonds, Keenan, Rohani, and Sachs, 2010; Boni, Galvani, Wickelgren, and Malani, 2013; Bonovas and Nikolopoulos, 2012). Over the centuries, Europeans had developed high degrees of herd immunity to these diseases, while the indigenous peoples had no such immunity (Oleś, Gudowska-Nowak, and Kleczkowski, 2012; Otte, Nugent, and McLeod, 2004; Ozawa, Portnoy, Getaneh, Clark, Knoll, Bishai, and Patwardhan, 2016).

Smallpox devastated the native population of Australia, killing around 50% of Indigenous Australians in the early years of British colonization (Armelagos, Brown, and Turner, 2005; Arokiasamy and Krishnan, 1994; Arora, 2001, 2005; Arredondo and Zúñiga, 2004). It also killed many New Zealand Māori (Bwire, Munier, Ouedraogo, Heyerdahl, Komakech, Kagirita, and Makumbi, 2017; Canali, Aragrande, Angheben, Capelli, Drigo, Gobbi, and Cassini, 2020). In 1848–49, as many as 40,000 out of 150,000 Hawaiians are estimated to have died of measles, whooping cough and influenza (Borghol, Suderman, McArdle, Racine, Hallett, Pembrey, and Szyf, 2012; Brandes, 2008; Brown, Lipscomb, and Snyder, 2001). Introduced diseases, notably smallpox, nearly wiped out the native population of Easter Island. Measles killed more than 40,000 Fijians, approximately one-third of the population, in 1875 (Peckham, 2013; Perrings et al., 2002, 2014). In the early 19th century, measles also devastated the Andamanese population (Amuna and Zotor, 2008; Aral, Holmes, Padian, and Cates, 1996; Arbabi, Nezami, Hooshyar, and Delavari, 2018). The Ainu population decreased drastically in the 19th century, due in large part to infectious diseases brought by Japanese settlers pouring into Hokkaido (Acemoglu and Johnson, 2007; Adda, 2016; Alloul, Sauriol, Kennedy, Laurier, Tessier, Novosel, and Contandriopoulos, 1998).

Researchers concluded that syphilis was carried from the New World to Europe after Columbus's voyages (Moné, Ibikounlé, Massougbodji, and Mouahid, 2010; Morand, 2004; Moro, Budke, Schantz, Vasquez, Santivanez, and Villavicencio, 2011). The findings suggested Europeans could have carried the non-venereal tropical bacteria home, where the organisms may have mutated into a deadlier form in the different conditions of Europe (Uusküla, Müürsepp, Kawai, Raag, Jürisson, and Pillsbury, 2013; Vanni, Karnon, Madan, White, Edmunds, Foss, and Legood, 2011). The disease was more frequently fatal than it is today (Raut, 2004; Rehm, Mathers, Popova, Thavorncharoensap, Teerawattananon, and Patra, 2009; Rich and Perry, 2011). Syphilis was a major killer in Europe during the Renaissance (Foxman, 2002; Garner, Whan, Gard, and Phillips, 2001; Gayle and Hill,

2001; Gottstein, Pozio, and Nöckler, 2009). Between 1602 and 1796, the Dutch East India Company sent almost a million Europeans to work in Asia (Howe, Häsler, and Stärk, 2013; Howe et al., 2012). Ultimately, fewer than a third made their way back to Europe (Weycker, Edelsberg, Oster, and Tino, 2005; Wu, Perrings, Kinzig, Collins, Minteer, and Daszak, 2017; Yach, Stuckler, and Brownell, 2006). The majority died of diseases. Disease killed more British soldiers in India and South Africa than war (Daily, and Ehrlich, 1996; Deogaonkar, Hutubessy, Van Der Putten, Evers, and Jit, 2012; Dorn, 1992; Ducrotoy, Bertu, Ocholi, Gusi, Bryssinckx, Welburn, and Moriyon, 2014).

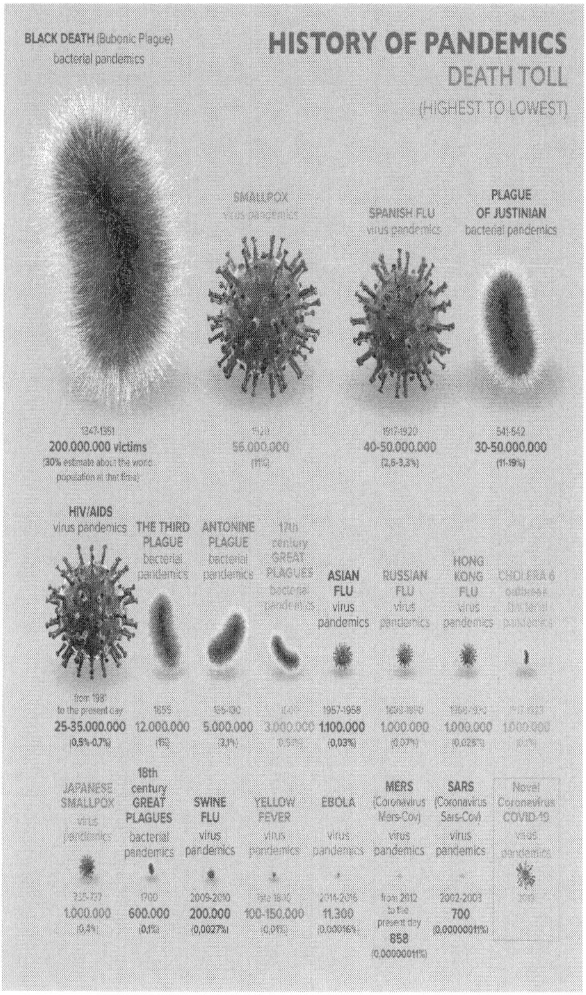

Source: https://www.shutterstock.com/

As early as 1803, the Spanish Crown organized a mission (the Balmis expedition) to transport the smallpox vaccine to the Spanish colonies, and establish mass vaccination programs there (Chen, Li, Hsieh, Chang, Lee, Lee, and Ko, 2012; Conover, Pitt, Kessler, DuBow, and Sanborn, 1995; Crump, Murdoch, and Baker, 2001). By 1832, the federal government of the United States established a smallpox vaccination program for Native Americans (Arredondo and Zúñiga, 2006; Backer, van Roermund, Fischer, van Asseldonk, and Bergevoet, 2015; Bartsch, Hotez, Hertenstein, Diemert, Zapf, Bottazzi, and Lee, 2016). From the beginning of the 20th century onwards, the elimination or control of disease in tropical countries became a driving force for all colonial powers (Rogers, Carolin, Vaught, and Compton, 2011; Ronohardjo and Rastiko, 1982; Sachs, 2001; Sachs and Malaney, 2002). The sleeping sickness epidemic in Africa was arrested due to mobile teams systematically screening millions of people at risk (Yi-Xin and Manderson, 2005; Zadoks, 2008; Zhan, Li, Wang, Sun, Geng, Xiong, and de Hoog, 2015; Zhang, Song, Cai, and Zhou, 2008). In the 20th century, the world saw the biggest increase in its population in human history due to a drop in the mortality rate in many countries as a result of medical advances (Perry and Randolph, 1999; Philipson, 2000; Philipson and Posner, 1996; Pongchaiyakul, Songpattanasilp, and Taechakraichana, 2008). The world population has grown from 1.6 billion in 1900 to an estimated 6.8 billion in 2011 and continues to grow (Abegunde and Stanciole, 2008; Abramowitz, Lacau Saint Guily, Moyal-Barracco, Bergeron, Borne, Dahlab, and Bénard, 2018). Even the COVID-19 pandemic has not yet been able to significantly reduce the global population, certainly not to the levels of 50% that were experienced in the past (Fenichel, 2013; Fenichel et al., 2011; Fogel, 1994). The final section in this chapter will summarize the economic impact of disease epidemics as an introduction to a later exploration of all the relevant social-economic indicators of decline following a disease epidemic.

1.5. THE ECONOMIC IMPACT OF DISEASE EPIDEMICS

Existing literature has established links between income and infectious disease epidemics. Researchers are particularly interested in how such links are affected by changing global circumstances (Saleha, 1991; Sibert, Rigaud, Delavierre, and Labat, 2010; Skrepnek and Skrepnek, 2004; Sloane, 2009; Sockett, 1993). In general, having money and living in a prosperous society protects individuals against health setbacks and epidemics (Bausch and Schwarz, 2014; Bausch et al., 2001; Benner, Carabin, Sánchez-Serrano, Budke, and Carmena, 2010). Healthy people get more education, are more productive in the workforce, attract foreign investment, and save more (Hart and Halden, 2020; Häsler, Howe, and Stärk, 2011; Henschke, Kamper, and Maher, 2015; Hochberg, 1992). As better health leads to decreases in family size, the consequent change in a country's age structure can boost economic growth (Ozmen, Kurşun, and Ozcelik, 2005; Paarlberg, Hillberg, Lee, and Mathews, 2008; Paisley, Vraa-Andersen, Dybkjaer, Møller, Christensen, Mousing, and Agger, 1993). In Figure 1.5, we see that the COVID-19 epidemic has had a somewhat negative impact on the markets, even if some areas are still doing fairly well. This shows that the adverse effects of disease pandemics are not always evenly distributed or even reflected accurately in the financial market positions in the short run (Buckley, 1984; Budke, Jiamin, Qian, and Torgerson, 2005; Bundy, Arámbulo III, and Grey, 1983; Buzby and Roberts, 2009). However, in the long run epidemics generally lead to falling economic growth indicators (Pal, Kerorsa, Marami, and Kandi, 2020; Paterson, Otte, Slingenbergh, Wint, and Rogers, 2000; Pearce and Merletti, 2006).

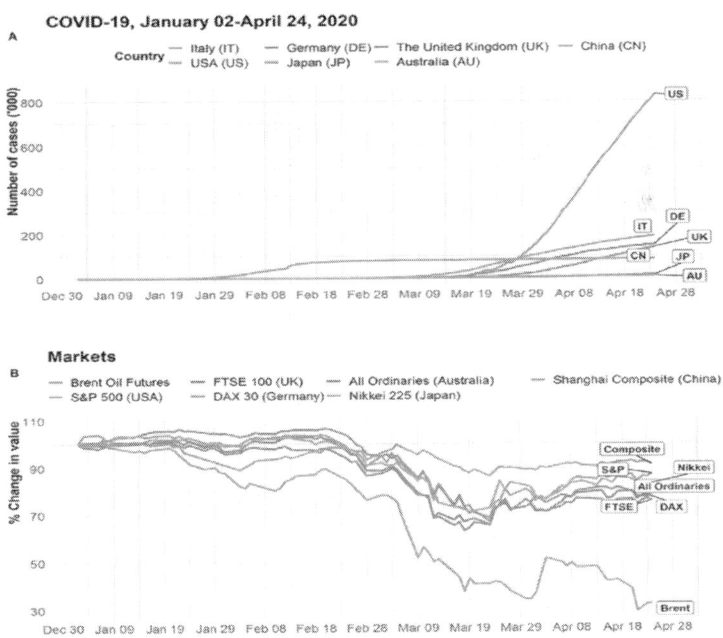

Figure 1.5. Economic consequences of COVID-19 outbreak.

Source: Frontiers.

Epidemics can dampen some of these effects by changing expectations about how well an economy will function and also by deterring investment and tourism (Narrod, Zinsstag, and Tiongco, 2012; Nascimento and de Oliveira, 2014; O'Brien, Lahue, Caro, and Davidson, 2007). For many countries, the immediate costs of an epidemic are apparent, while the long-term costs are less obvious (Krieger, 2001a, b; Lemma, 1969; Liu, Maniadakis, Gray, and Rayner, 2002; López, Torné, Franco, San-Martin, Viayna, Barrull, and Perulero, 2018). Nevertheless, when accounting for the value of human life in the cost, epidemics become significantly costly (Jenkins, Baingana, Ahmad, McDaid, and Atun, 2011; Johnson, Alvarez-Pasquin, Bijl, Franco, Gaillat, Clara, and Weinke, 2015). Preventing epidemics requires overcoming obstacles (Purevdawa, Moon, Baigalmaa, Davaajav, Smith, and Vermund, 1997; Ramesh, Malla, Raju, Sehgal, Ganguly, Mahajan, and Dilawari, 1990). Similarly, resources are expended in responding to an epidemic once it begins (Purevdawa, Moon, Baigalmaa, Davaajav, Smith, and Vermund, 1997; Ramesh, Malla, Raju, Sehgal, Ganguly, Mahajan, and Dilawari, 1990). Globally, long-term vulnerability to epidemics may decrease as development standards rise, but a more highly interconnected world may actually promote the occurrence of infectious disease epidemics(Jenkins, Baingana, Ahmad, McDaid, and Atun, 2011; Johnson, Alvarez-Pasquin, Bijl, Franco, Gaillat, Clara, and Weinke, 2015).

The association between health and wealth is well established in existing literature (Krieger, 2001a, b; Lemma, 1969; Liu, Maniadakis, Gray, and Rayner, 2002; López, Torné, Franco, San-Martin, Viayna, Barrull, and Perulero, 2018). Wealthier countries tend to generally have healthier populations than poor countries (Narrod, Zinsstag, and Tiongco, 2012; Nascimento and de Oliveira, 2014; O'Brien, Lahue, Caro, and Davidson, 2007). For example, life expectancy increases sharply as income per capita rises among poorer countries and continues to rise, though at a much slower rate, as countries become wealthier (Pal, Kerorsa, Marami, and Kandi, 2020; Paterson, Otte, Slingenbergh, Wint, and Rogers, 2000; Pearce and Merletti, 2006). Between 1995 and 2000, life expectancy at birth in the world's least developed countries was 51 years (Buckley, 1984; Budke, Jiamin, Qian, and Torgerson, 2005; Bundy, Arámbulo III, and Grey, 1983; Buzby and Roberts, 2009). In other low-income countries it was 59 years, in middle-income countries 70 years, and in high-income countries 78 years (Ozmen, Kurşun, and Ozcelik, 2005; Paarlberg, Hillberg, Lee, and Mathews, 2008; Paisley, Vraa-Andersen, Dybkjaer, Møller, Christensen, Mousing, and Agger, 1993). For a long period of time, it was assumed that the causality ran in only one direction whereby health improved as in-comes rose (Hart and Halden, 2020; Häsler, Howe, and Stärk, 2011; Henschke, Kamper, and Maher, 2015; Hochberg, 1992). More recently, researchers have identified a more nuanced view of these variables. For example, we have seen increased attention paid to assessing the reverse effects, as health has come to be seen as a key driver of economic development (Bausch and Schwarz, 2014; Bausch et al., 2001; Benner, Carabin, Sánchez-Serrano, Budke, and Carmena, 2010).

The view that higher incomes lead to better health stems from several mechanisms (Saleha, 1991; Sibert, Rigaud, Delavierre, and Labat, 2010; Skrepnek and Skrepnek, 2004; Sloane, 2009; Sockett, 1993). For example, wealthier individuals within a population can afford the essential products necessary for a healthy life (Fenichel, 2013; Fenichel et al., 2011; Fogel, 1994). For instance, they will have sufficient, nutritious food, adequate housing, clean water, and quality health care as a starting point (Abegunde and Stanciole, 2008; Abramowitz, Lacau Saint Guily, Moyal-Barracco, Bergeron, Borne, Dahlab, and Bénard, 2018). Moreover, wealthier people have better access to information and therefore have more knowledge of how to foster and maintain their health (Perry and Randolph, 1999; Philipson, 2000; Philipson and Posner, 1996; Pongchaiyakul, Songpattanasilp, and Taechakraichana, 2008). The wealthy have a stronger influence with policymakers than the poor, so their demands for improvements in health services are more likely to be acted upon (Yi-Xin and Manderson, 2005; Zadoks, 2008; Zhan, Li, Wang, Sun, Geng, Xiong, and de Hoog, 2015; Zhang, Song, Cai, and Zhou, 2008). Wealthier countries and their residents enjoy resilience-building advantages in education, ability to develop and buy medicines and other health technologies, training, and paying doctors and nurses, building, and maintaining hospitals and clinics, and minimizing nosocomial infections (Rogers, Carolin, Vaught, and Compton, 2011; Ronohardjo and Rastiko, 1982; Sachs, 2001; Sachs and Malaney, 2002). Wealthier nations also excel in providing water and sanitation facilities, using less noxious energy sources, and implementing comprehensive public health campaigns (Arredondo and Zúñiga, 2006; Backer, van Roermund, Fischer, van Asseldonk, and Bergevoet, 2015; Bartsch, Hotez, Hertenstein, Diemert, Zapf, Bottazzi, and Lee, 2016).

Ultimately, it is the poor (particularly the urban poor) that suffer most from disease epidemics (Chen, Li, Hsieh, Chang, Lee, Lee, and Ko, 2012; Conover, Pitt, Kessler, DuBow, and Sanborn, 1995; Crump, Murdoch, and Baker, 2001). Their crowded living conditions are ideal grounds for diseases to emerge and spread rapidly. Urbanization gives the semblance of development whilst masking an underclass of people who are living on the margins of a seemingly affluent society (Daily, and Ehrlich, 1996; Deogaonkar, Hutubessy, Van Der Putten, Evers, and Jit, 2012; Dorn, 1992; Ducrotoy, Bertu, Ocholi, Gusi, Bryssinckx, Welburn, and Moriyon, 2014). Indeed, this is one of the problems that have been identified in developed nations which otherwise seem to be thriving (Weycker, Edelsberg, Oster, and Tino, 2005; Wu, Perrings, Kinzig, Collins, Minteer, and Daszak, 2017; Yach, Stuckler, and Brownell, 2006). Yet, a close examination will reveal significant inequalities that increase their vulnerabilities to deadly pandemics (Howe, Häsler, and Stärk, 2013; Howe et al., 2012). COVID-19 has significantly impacted on the developed world, but interestingly it is the poor and ethnic minorities that are bearing the brunt of case fatalities (Foxman, 2002; Garner, Whan, Gard, and Phillips, 2001; Gayle and Hill, 2001; Gottstein, Pozio, and Nöckler, 2009). The wealthy tend to have better lifestyles which give them resilience and a greater opportunity for recovery (Raut, 2004; Rehm, Mathers, Popova, Thavorncharoensap, Teerawattananon, and Patra, 2009; Rich and Perry, 2011).

Health is a key element when creating a thriving, productive society (Uusküla, Müürsepp, Kawai, Raag, Jürisson, and Pillsbury, 2013; Vanni, Karnon, Madan, White, Edmunds, Foss, and Legood, 2011) (Moné, Ibikounlé, Massougbodji, and Mouahid, 2010; Morand, 2004; Moro, Budke, Schantz, Vasquez, Santivanez, and Villavicencio, 2011). However, fear, and illness can stifle production, consumption, recreation, travel, and overall well-being (Tapia, 2003; Torgerson and Dowling, 2001; Torgerson, Carmona, and Bonifacino, 2000; Uddin Khan, Atanasova, Krueger, Ramirez, and Gray, 2013). We have already seen this in the COVID-19 crises where many otherwise prosperous economies have faced recession and retreat due to fears of infection. While sectors outside of health are often considered in the context of negative externalities in driving disease events, the potential impacts they face from disease events warrants their engagement in finding multi-sectoral solutions to reduce and manage disease risks (Bergevoet, Van Schaik, Veling, Backus, and Franken, 2009; Binder, 1988; Bolos, Bacarea, and Marusteri, 2011). On a broad scale, far-reaching impacts of pandemics parallel other disasters (Suhrcke, Stuckler, Suk, Desai, Senek, McKee, and Rechel, 2011; Šumilo, Bormane, Asokliene, Vasilenko, Golovljova, Avsic-Zupanc, and Randolph, 2008). The Ebola epidemic in West Africa, for example, demonstrated the serious, and unanticipated, economic toll of an emerging infectious disease (Markos and Abdela, 2016; Martin and Shepherd, 2009; McGuinness, McGlynn, Johnson, MacIntyre, Batty, Burns, and McGinty, 2012). From 2013 to 2014, gross domestic product (GDP) growth in Liberia decreased from 8.7% to 0.7%, due to Ebola and lowering commodity prices, and GDP growth in Sierra Leone (with the exception of iron ore) decreased from 5.3% to 0.8% (Espinoza, Terashima, Herrera-Velit, and Marcos, 2010; Ezzati, Vander Hoorn, Lawes, Leach, James, Lopez, and Murray, 2005). GDP growth in Guinea in 2015, predicted at 4%, fell to 0.1% (Eaton and Groopman, 2013; Eckelman, Sherman, and MacNeill, 2018; Egger, 2011; Elbe, 2007; Ernst and Hay, 1994). In all three countries, government revenues declined across the board, including direct taxes on companies, VAT receipts, and indirect taxes (Acemoglu and Johnson, 2007; Adda, 2016; Alloul, Sauriol, Kennedy, Laurier, Tessier, Novosel, and Contandriopoulos, 1998). Additionally, the decline in private and foreign investors' confidence led to financing gaps of more than US $600 million over the 2 years.

These impacts cut across many sectors and undoubtedly have long-term consequences, including implications for insurers and reinsurers as well as overall business continuity from lack of worker capacity during illness (Amuna and Zotor, 2008; Aral, Holmes, Padian, and Cates, 1996; Arbabi, Nezami, Hooshyar, and Delavari, 2018). However, there are markets which are emerging to ensure against pandemic risk (Peckham, 2013; Perrings et al., 2002, 2014). Examples include the World Bank's Pandemic Emergency Financing Facility (Borghol, Suderman, McArdle, Racine, Hallett, Pembrey, and Szyf, 2012; Brandes, 2008; Brown, Lipscomb, and Snyder, 2001). This is a parametric insurance vehicle designed to provide rapid disbursement of emergency finance (Bwire, Munier, Ouedraogo, Heyerdahl, Komakech, Kagirita, and Makumbi, 2017; Canali, Aragrande, Angheben, Capelli, Drigo, Gobbi, and Cassini, 2020). Yet engagement of the private sector, as well as public institutions beyond the health sector, remains limited in overall epidemic and pandemic planning and intervention (Armelagos, Brown, and Turner, 2005; Arokiasamy and Krishnan, 1994; Arora, 2001, 2005; Arredondo and Zúñiga, 2004). Given the reality of pandemics and the risk of them increasing due to population growth and urbanization, it makes sense for governments to put contingency plans in place (Oleś, Gudowska-Nowak, and Kleczkowski, 2012; Otte, Nugent, and McLeod, 2004; Ozawa, Portnoy, Getaneh, Clark, Knoll, Bishai, and Patwardhan, 2016).

CHAPTER 1 SUMMARY

This introductory chapter has summarized the nature of epidemics in terms of their spread, spatial scope, and timelines. The chapter has also introduced examples of notorious epidemics as identified by their high rates of fatality cases. In doing so, the chapter has shown the vulnerabilities of poor and urban populations to these outbreaks. Finally, the chapter identified some of the economic implications of epidemics and pandemics. In the next chapter, we will consider the origins and drivers of disease epidemics.

Chapter

2 Origins and Drivers of Disease Epidemics

CONTENTS

Those who are responsible for preventing and responding to disease epidemics would prefer a preventative approach. This requires a proactive view of the causes and drivers of disease epidemics so that they can be controlled or neutralized. This chapter explores some of those causes in terms of ecological changes, human population growth, cultural practices, lifestyle changes, and the rather conspiracy-driven notion of bio-weaponry. By the end of this chapter, the reader should have a broad understanding of how these factors contribute to the outbreak of disease epidemics. In so doing, the chapter providers additional insights into how certain disease epidemics can be minimized, if not prevented completely.

2.1. CHANGES IN THE ECOLOGY AND DISEASE EPIDEMICS

Environmental changes have a huge impact on the emergence and re-emergence of certain infectious diseases (Bonds, Keenan, Rohani, and Sachs, 2010; Boni, Galvani, Wickelgren, and Malani, 2013; Bonovas and Nikolopoulos, 2012). This occurs mainly in countries with high biodiversity and serious unresolved environmental, social, and economic issues (Kim and Goldie, 2008; Klein, Laxminarayan, Smith, and Gilligan, 2007; Klepac, Laxminarayan, and Grenfell, 2011). A case in point is Brazil where there are a number of diseases, these present public health challenges, notably stemming from the likes of Chikungunya, dengue fever, yellow fever, Zika, hantavirus pulmonary syndrome, leptospirosis, leishmaniasis, and Chagas disease (St George, 1986; Steben and Duarte-Franco, 2007; Stehr-Green and Schantz, 1987; Stuckler, 2008; Stuckler and Siegel, 2011). There is a relationship between infectious diseases outbreaks and climate change events (Poundstone, Strathdee, and Celentano, 2004; Pritchett, Thilmany, and Johnson, 2005; Pugliatti, Beghi, Forsgren, Ekman, and Sobocki, 2007).

Some of the key event cited in existing literature include El Niño, La Niña, heatwaves, droughts, floods, increased temperature, and higher rainfall (Casamassimo, Thikkurissy, Edelstein, and Maiorini, 2009; Castro, Wilson, and Bloom, 2017). Another causative factor may be environmental changes such as habitat fragmentation, deforestation, urbanization, and bushmeat consumption (Yi-Xin and Manderson, 2005; Zadoks, 2008; Zhan, Li, Wang, Sun, Geng, Xiong, and de Hoog, 2015; Zhang, Song, Cai, and Zhou, 2008). To avoid or control outbreaks, integrated surveillance systems and effective outreach programs are essential (Weycker, Edelsberg, Oster, and Tino, 2005; Wu, Perrings, Kinzig, Collins, Minteer, and Daszak, 2017; Yach,

Stuckler, and Brownell, 2006). Due to strong global and local influence on the emergence of infectious diseases, a more holistic approach is necessary to mitigate or control them in low-income nations (Uusküla, Müürsepp, Kawai, Raag, Jürisson, and Pillsbury, 2013; Vanni, Karnon, Madan, White, Edmunds, Foss, and Legood, 2011). Sometimes these disease epidemics become part of a much wider pattern of disruptions on the global economy (see Figure 2.1). Hence, the urgency of identifying their causes, drivers, and possible solutions (Tapia, 2003; Torgerson and Dowling, 2001; Torgerson, Carmona, and Bonifacino, 2000; Uddin Khan, Atanasova, Krueger, Ramirez, and Gray, 2013).

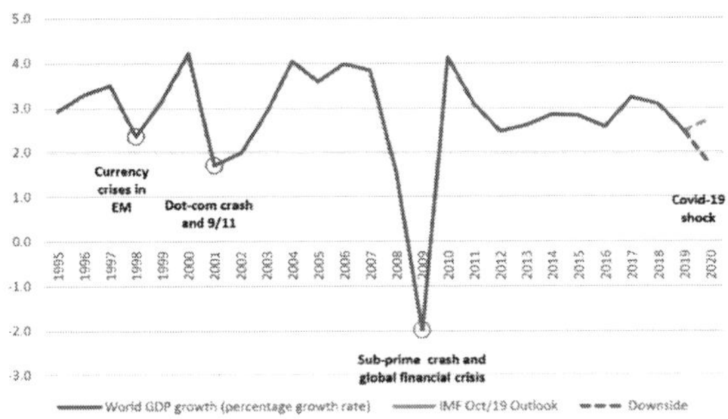

Figure 2.1. Economic impact of COVID-19 pandemic.

Source: UNIDO.

It is widely accepted that human modifications to the environment are the main causes or drivers for global environmental changes (Suhrcke, Stuckler, Suk, Desai, Senek, McKee, and Rechel, 2011; Šumilo, Bormane, Asokliene, Vasilenko, Golovljova, Avsic-Zupanc, and Randolph, 2008). Indeed, some researchers state that global environmental change is both systemic and cumulative (St George, 1986; Steben and Duarte-Franco, 2007; Stehr-Green and Schantz, 1987; Stuckler, 2008; Stuckler and Siegel, 2011). Diverse scientific fields have generated enormous data about the complex environmental systems on our planet with conclusive evidence of anthropogenic environmental change (Saleha, 1991; Sibert, Rigaud, Delavierre, and Labat, 2010; Skrepnek and Skrepnek, 2004; Sloane, 2009; Sockett, 1993). Some authors have proposed that due to human-induced global environmental changes, planet Earth has entered a new geological epoch termed the Anthropocene (Rogers, Carolin, Vaught, and Compton, 2011; Ronohardjo and Rastiko, 1982; Sachs, 2001; Sachs and Malaney, 2002). Building on the Millennium Ecosystem Assessment definition of drivers of ecosystem change, researchers define drivers of ecosystem change as a complex web of interactions between humans and their surroundings as humans seek to satisfy their basic needs and improve their wellbeing (Raut, 2004; Rehm, Mathers, Popova, Thavorncharoensap, Teerawattananon, and Patra, 2009; Rich and Perry, 2011). There are many anthropogenic drivers of environmental changes and they are the result of development and economic pressures (Purevdawa, Moon, Baigalmaa, Davaajav, Smith, and Vermund, 1997; Ramesh, Malla, Raju, Sehgal, Ganguly, Mahajan, and Dilawari, 1990).

According to the World Health Organization (WHO), environmental threats to human health at global and regional levels include: climate change, stratospheric ozone depletion, changes in ecosystems due to loss of biodiversity, changes in hydrological systems and supplies of fresh water, land degradation, urbanization, and stresses on food-producing systems (Poundstone, Strathdee, and Celentano, 2004; Pritchett, Thilmany, and Johnson, 2005; Pugliatti, Beghi, Forsgren, Ekman, and Sobocki, 2007). Rapid social and environmental changes are occurring globally, affecting both low-income countries and the largest advanced economies (Perry and Randolph, 1999; Philipson, 2000; Philipson and Posner, 1996; Pongchaiyakul, Songpattanasilp, and Taechakraichana, 2008). Travel and transportation are the greatest increase to the risks of rapid spread of infectious diseases (Peckham, 2013; Perrings et al., 2002, 2014). This is particularly true in the tropics where there is high biodiversity and where ecological change is greatest (Pal, Kerorsa, Marami, and Kandi, 2020; Paterson, Otte, Slingenbergh, Wint, and Rogers, 2000; Pearce and Merletti, 2006). Hence, these regions have become potential hotspots for the emergence of new pathogens affecting human, wildlife, and domestic animal health (Ozmen, Kurşun, and Ozcelik, 2005; Paarlberg, Hillberg, Lee, and Mathews, 2008; Paisley, Vraa-Andersen, Dybkjaer, Møller, Christensen, Mousing, and Agger, 1993).

Emerging infectious diseases are increasingly recognized as a global threat, with major concerns on their rapid global spread (Moné, Ibikounlé, Massougbodji, and Mouahid, 2010; Morand, 2004; Moro, Budke, Schantz, Vasquez, Santivanez, and Villavicencio, 2011). To effectively design prevention and control programs, the complex and fluid relationships among multi-host and multi-pathogen systems, environmental change, and human populations must be thoroughly understood (Markos and Abdela, 2016; Martin and Shepherd, 2009; McGuinness, McGlynn, Johnson, MacIntyre, Batty, Burns, and McGinty, 2012). Improved and targeted surveillance systems will provide better knowledge for analysis of the specific risks of disease emergence (Krieger, 2001a, b; Lemma, 1969; Liu, Maniadakis, Gray, and Rayner, 2002; López, Torné, Franco, San-Martin, Viayna, Barrull, and Perulero, 2018). The interactions among wildlife, domestic animals, and humans can exist in different landscapes and are implicated as potential causes of important outbreaks globally (Kim and Goldie, 2008; Klein, Laxminarayan, Smith, and Gilligan, 2007; Klepac, Laxminarayan, and Grenfell, 2011). Host-pathogen interactions can be strongly affected by species diversity and community composition (Jenkins, Baingana, Ahmad, McDaid, and Atun, 2011; Johnson, Alvarez-Pasquin, Bijl, Franco, Gaillat, Clara, and Weinke, 2015). Therefore, it is urgently necessary to understand the effects of habitat fragmentation and other environmental changes on host-pathogen interactions (Howe, Häsler, and Stärk, 2013; Howe et al., 2012). Establishing local policies that require integrated assessments prior to development projects can help predict risks and emphasize practices to mitigate the disease transmission between humans and other species (Hart and Halden, 2020; Häsler, Howe, and Stärk, 2011; Henschke, Kamper, and Maher, 2015; Hochberg, 1992). The next section examines how the human population grows drives disease epidemics and makes them difficult to control when they eventually occur.

2.2. HUMAN POPULATION GROWTH AND DISEASE EPIDEMICS

Existing literature has shown that in many ways and to various extents, population growth drives infectious disease rate upward (Foxman, 2002; Garner, Whan, Gard, and Phillips, 2001; Gayle and Hill, 2001; Gottstein, Pozio, and Nöckler, 2009). For example, demand-driven agriculture and livestock production are predicted to increase the spread and dangers of zoonotic diseases (Fenichel, 2013; Fenichel et al., 2011; Fogel, 1994). As the world population grows, the rise of mega agriculture to meet increased demand for food could aid the spread and virulence of infectious diseases worldwide (Espinoza, Terashima, Herrera-Velit, and Marcos, 2010; Ezzati, Vander Hoorn, Lawes, Leach, James, Lopez, and Murray, 2005). Developing nations, where most of the population growth is expected to occur, will race to meet the demands, but poor public health infrastructures could put the global food supply at risk (Eaton and Groopman, 2013; Eckelman, Sherman, and MacNeill, 2018; Egger, 2011; Elbe, 2007; Ernst and Hay, 1994). In the next decades, we will see significant global, societal, and agricultural shifts in what has been dubbed "The Next Food Revolution" (Daily, and Ehrlich,

1996; Deogaonkar, Hutubessy, Van Der Putten, Evers, and Jit, 2012; Dorn, 1992; Ducrotoy, Bertu, Ocholi, Gusi, Bryssinckx, Welburn, and Moriyon, 2014). The revolution will include numerous opportunities for already well-adaptable microbes (Chen, Li, Hsieh, Chang, Lee, Lee, and Ko, 2012; Conover, Pitt, Kessler, DuBow, and Sanborn, 1995; Crump, Murdoch, and Baker, 2001). As we see in Figure 2.2, the people who will be the most negatively affected by disease epidemics will be those that are living in the developing world.

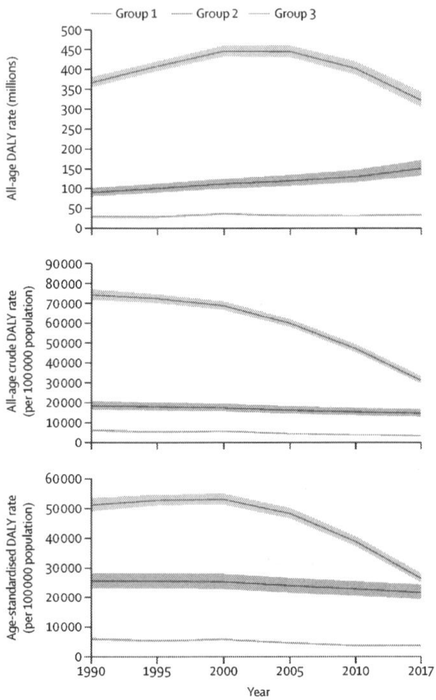

Figure 2.2. Burden of non-communicable diseases in sub-Saharan Africa.

Source: The Lancet.

Some refer to this as a perfect microbial storm where the winners are the microbes who change, move, and cross-species lines and acquire resistance (Casamassimo, Thikkurissy, Edelstein, and Maiorini, 2009; Castro, Wilson, and Bloom, 2017). Three eras should be considered when examining public health solutions to the spread of zoonotic diseases (Bwire, Munier, Ouedraogo, Heyerdahl, Komakech, Kagirita, and Makumbi, 2017; Canali, Aragrande, Angheben, Capelli, Drigo, Gobbi, and Cassini, 2020).

The advent of agriculture was the first contributor to the problem (Buckley, 1984; Budke, Jiamin, Qian, and Torgerson, 2005; Bundy, Arámbulo III, and Grey, 1983; Buzby and Roberts, 2009). When humans started to grow their own food, they remained stable and built communities (Borghol, Suderman, McArdle, Racine, Hallett, Pembrey, and Szyf, 2012; Brandes, 2008; Brown, Lipscomb, and Snyder, 2001). Consequently, infectious diseases were able to spread and grow in these stable human populations (Bonds, Keenan, Rohani, and Sachs, 2010; Boni, Galvani, Wickelgren, and Malani, 2013; Bonovas and Nikolopoulos, 2012). Animal domestication marks the second zoonotic era (Bergevoet, Van Schaik, Veling, Backus, and Franken, 2009; Binder, 1988; Bolos, Bacarea, and Marusteri, 2011). The first zoonotic seasons likely began as humans began living with animals that were raised as livestock (Bausch and Schwarz, 2014; Bausch et al., 2001; Benner, Carabin, Sánchez-Serrano, Budke, and Carmena, 2010). A third transition occurred in the last 25 to 35 years (Arredondo and Zúñiga, 2006; Backer, van Roermund, Fischer, van Asseldonk, and Bergevoet, 2015; Bartsch, Hotez, Hertenstein, Diemert, Zapf, Bottazzi, and Lee, 2016). This was characterized by newly emerging infectious diseases and conditions that created a new world in which 75% of major infectious diseases were zoonotic (Armelagos, Brown, and Turner, 2005; Arokiasamy and Krishnan, 1994; Arora, 2001, 2005; Arredondo and Zúñiga, 2004). Factors contributing to the perfect storm include microbial adaption to change and susceptibility, climate, weather, and changing ecosystems (Amuna and Zotor, 2008; Aral, Holmes, Padian, and Cates, 1996; Arbabi, Nezami, Hooshyar, and Delavari, 2018).

Technology and industry also facilitated the spread of microbes to more populations in less time (Acemoglu and Johnson, 2007; Adda, 2016; Alloul, Sauriol, Kennedy, Laurier, Tessier, Novosel, and Contandriopoulos, 1998). Some estimates indicate that on an annual basis, up to 1.5 million people are traveling internationally, and they help to spread diseases much like the recent COVID-19 outbreak (Abegunde and Stanciole, 2008; Abramowitz, Lacau Saint Guily, Moyal-Barracco, Bergeron, Borne, Dahlab, and Bénard, 2018). The microbes are the winners, changing, adapting, acquiring resistance and moving worldwide (Ozmen, Kurşun, and Ozcelik, 2005; Paarlberg, Hillberg, Lee, and Mathews, 2008; Paisley, Vraa-Andersen, Dybkjaer, Møller, Christensen, Mousing, and Agger, 1993). They are doing well in ways that are unprecedented according to some experts since they are exposed to a wide diversity of populations through modern travel (Bonds, Keenan, Rohani, and Sachs, 2010; Boni, Galvani, Wickelgren, and Malani, 2013; Bonovas and Nikolopoulos, 2012). The growth and the shift of populations from rural to urban farming are a driving force behind the need for food and the need to closely monitor production (Espinoza, Terashima, Herrera-Velit, and Marcos, 2010; Ezzati, Vander Hoorn, Lawes, Leach, James, Lopez, and Murray, 2005). The demand to feed the planet's 7 billion people is driving food production from industrialized to developing nations (Buckley, 1984; Budke, Jiamin, Qian, and Torgerson, 2005; Bundy, Arámbulo III, and Grey, 1983; Buzby and Roberts, 2009).

By 2015, more than 90% of the world's population growth was in developing nations, which may lack the infrastructure to thwart zoonotic and foodborne diseases (Bwire, Munier, Ouedraogo, Heyerdahl, Komakech, Kagirita, and Makumbi, 2017; Canali, Aragrande, Angheben, Capelli, Drigo, Gobbi, and Cassini, 2020). These nations are potential hot spots for new emerging diseases and have been the centers of epidemics in the past such as HIV/AIDS and Ebola (Yi-Xin and Manderson, 2005; Zadoks, 2008; Zhan, Li, Wang, Sun, Geng, Xiong, and de Hoog, 2015; Zhang, Song, Cai, and Zhou, 2008). Shifts from rural farming to urban farming are also areas of concern (Pal, Kerorsa, Marami, and Kandi, 2020; Paterson, Otte, Slingenbergh, Wint, and Rogers, 2000; Pearce and Merletti, 2006). In 2030, an estimated 60% of people will live in urban areas (Jenkins, Baingana, Ahmad, McDaid, and Atun, 2011; Johnson, Alvarez-Pasquin, Bijl, Franco, Gaillat, Clara, and Weinke, 2015). Infectious and zoonotic diseases will be harder to control because livestock farming is predicted to move to the edge of these urban areas (Abegunde and Stanciole, 2008; Abramowitz, Lacau Saint Guily, Moyal-Barracco, Bergeron, Borne, Dahlab, and Bénard, 2018). Animal production will boom in places that may lack in public health. Some have suggested that to feed billions of people, you have to concentrate the animals in a way that there are environments for the animals themselves (Kim and Goldie, 2008; Klein, Laxminarayan, Smith, and Gilligan, 2007; Klepac, Laxminarayan, and Grenfell, 2011). Hence, animal farming is already to the point where an egg can grow to a full-grown bird in 41 days for production purposes as a case in point (Chen, Li, Hsieh, Chang, Lee, Lee, and Ko, 2012; Conover, Pitt, Kessler, DuBow, and Sanborn, 1995; Crump, Murdoch, and Baker, 2001). In the United States, the annual burden of foodborne illness is 76 million illnesses, 25,000 hospitalizations, and 5,000 deaths (Weycker, Edelsberg, Oster, and Tino, 2005; Wu, Perrings, Kinzig, Collins, Minteer, and Daszak, 2017; Yach, Stuckler, and Brownell, 2006). The bulk of common foodborne pathogens are zoonotic and can be communicable (Perry and Randolph, 1999; Philipson, 2000; Philipson and Posner, 1996; Pongchaiyakul, Songpattanasilp, and Taechakraichana, 2008).

Another factor of the phenomenon some experts are calling the largest agricultural evolution in history is a demand-driven population outsourcing more crops and vegetable production to developing nations (Uusküla, Müürsepp, Kawai, Raag, Jürisson, and Pillsbury, 2013; Vanni, Karnon, Madan, White, Edmunds, Foss, and Legood, 2011). Crop production can increase the population's wealth; in turn, people's lifestyles will change, as well, shifting many from poverty to a new type of middle class and Westernization (St George, 1986; Steben and Duarte-Franco, 2007; Stehr-Green and Schantz, 1987; Stuckler, 2008; Stuckler and Siegel, 2011). When the population progresses above the poverty level, the increased demand for animal protein will be massive (Acemoglu and Johnson, 2007; Adda, 2016; Alloul, Sauriol, Kennedy, Laurier, Tessier, Novosel, and Contandriopoulos, 1998). A current prediction is that there will be a 50% increase globally for animal protein by the year 2020 (Amuna and Zotor, 2008; Aral, Holmes, Padian, and Cates, 1996; Arbabi, Nezami, Hooshyar, and Delavari, 2018). Understanding how societal changes and the changes in animals and their environments affect microbes are important for initiating measures for safe food supplies (Krieger, 2001a, b; Lemma, 1969; Liu, Maniadakis, Gray, and Rayner, 2002; López, Torné, Franco, San-Martin, Viayna, Barrull, and Perulero, 2018). The impact of mega agricultural production on populations as they relate to infectious disease also must be considered (Armelagos, Brown, and Turner, 2005; Arokiasamy and Krishnan, 1994; Arora, 2001, 2005; Arredondo and Zúñiga, 2004).

As the developed world moves to importing more food from developing countries, problems with infectious disease related to food are anticipated (Poundstone, Strathdee, and Celentano, 2004; Pritchett, Thilmany, and Johnson, 2005; Pugliatti, Beghi, Forsgren, Ekman, and Sobocki, 2007). Good animal health strategies are public health strategies, although they are often considered separate entities (Suhrcke, Stuckler, Suk, Desai, Senek, McKee, and Rechel, 2011; Šumilo, Bormane, Asokliene, Vasilenko, Golovljova, Avsic-Zupanc, and Randolph, 2008). Zoonotic diseases are "equal-opportunity microbes," but they do not infect people equally. A major concern are health disparities in resource-limited countries (Bergevoet, Van Schaik, Veling, Backus, and Franken, 2009; Binder, 1988; Bolos, Bacarea, and Marusteri, 2011). Women and children will get infected at the highest levels because they traditionally care for livestock in developing nations (Arredondo and Zúñiga, 2006; Backer, van Roermund, Fischer, van Asseldonk, and Bergevoet, 2015; Bartsch, Hotez, Hertenstein, Diemert, Zapf, Bottazzi, and Lee, 2016). Shifts from rural livestock to farms closer to urban areas or the fringe of forests also have major implications for infectious diseases (Howe, Häsler, and Stärk, 2013; Howe et al., 2012). For example, fruit bat saliva dropping on hogs have led to entire herds being killed as a result of infectious diseases (Raut, 2004; Rehm, Mathers, Popova, Thavorncharoensap, Teerawattananon, and Patra, 2009; Rich and Perry, 2011).

As humans do not often come into contact with wildlife, such pathogens should theoretically not pose much danger to people (Hart and Halden, 2020; Häsler, Howe, and Stärk, 2011; Henschke, Kamper, and Maher, 2015; Hochberg, 1992). But the pathogens can make the leap to humans by first infecting other animals that humans do come into contact with, such as domestic pigs (Markos and Abdela, 2016; Martin and Shepherd, 2009; McGuinness, McGlynn, Johnson, MacIntyre, Batty, Burns, and McGinty, 2012). The animals serving as the middle link of this disease chain, however, have to be in places in some overlapping territory, which occurs when burgeoning populations push people into wild areas where humans once rarely, if ever, ventured (Foxman, 2002; Garner, Whan, Gard, and Phillips, 2001; Gayle and Hill, 2001; Gottstein, Pozio, and Nöckler, 2009). The number of pathogens originating in wildlife and infecting humans has increased with time. In the last decade of the 20th century, such pathogens were responsible for more than half of the new infectious diseases that cropped up in that time period (Moné, Ibikounlé, Massougbodji, and Mouahid, 2010; Morand, 2004; Moro, Budke, Schantz, Vasquez, Santivanez, and Villavicencio, 2011). Human contact with wildlife species that facilitate the transmission of novel viruses may increase in the future, as the population grows and humans searching for places to live and farm fan out to areas inhabited by or closer to wildlife (Eaton and Groopman, 2013; Eckelman, Sherman, and MacNeill, 2018; Egger, 2011; Elbe, 2007; Ernst and Hay, 1994).

It is generally expected that in developing countries the epidemiological transition, with improved health and lower mortality rates, will eventually lead to a demographic transition with lower fertility rates (Oleś, Gudowska-Nowak, and Kleczkowski, 2012; Otte, Nugent, and McLeod, 2004; Ozawa, Portnoy, Getaneh, Clark, Knoll, Bishai, and Patwardhan, 2016). The reductions in mortality characterizing the epidemiological transition are often associated with controlling the infectious diseases within populations (Rogers, Carolin, Vaught, and Compton, 2011; Ronohardjo and Rastiko, 1982; Sachs, 2001; Sachs and Malaney, 2002). This leaves the chronic diseases associated with old age, cancer, and heart disease dominating the causes of death (Bausch and Schwarz, 2014; Bausch et al., 2001; Benner,

Carabin, Sánchez-Serrano, Budke, and Carmena, 2010). However, if the demographic transition does not occur quickly, populations can grow rapidly, creating an increased potential for spread of infectious disease (Purevdawa, Moon, Baigalmaa, Davaajav, Smith, and Vermund, 1997; Ramesh, Malla, Raju, Sehgal, Ganguly, Mahajan, and Dilawari, 1990). These infectious diseases could, in turn, increase death rates amongst young people and reverse the epidemiological transition (Borghol, Suderman, McArdle, Racine, Hallett, Pembrey, and Szyf, 2012; Brandes, 2008; Brown, Lipscomb, and Snyder, 2001). The relationship between population growth, size, and infection depends upon the changes in contact pattern associated with there being more people (Tapia, 2003; Torgerson and Dowling, 2001; Torgerson, Carmona, and Bonifacino, 2000; Uddin Khan, Atanasova, Krueger, Ramirez, and Gray, 2013). If facilities can keep pace with growth, then the increase in contact rates can be kept to a minimum, and the potential reversal in the epidemic transition prevented (Saleha, 1991; Sibert, Rigaud, Delavierre, and Labat, 2010; Skrepnek and Skrepnek, 2004; Sloane, 2009; Sockett, 1993). This makes development a crucial adjunct to population growth if the global community is not to be increasingly exposed to pandemics of infectious disease (Peckham, 2013; Perrings et al., 2002, 2014). In the next chapter, we consider how cultural practices impact on disease epidemiology.

2.3. CULTURAL PRACTICES AND DISEASE EPIDEMICS

Cultural aspects have a great influence on the processes of symptom recognition, labeling, help-seeking, and the structure of health systems (Daily, and Ehrlich, 1996; Deogaonkar, Hutubessy, Van Der Putten, Evers, and Jit, 2012; Dorn, 1992; Ducrotoy, Bertu, Ocholi, Gusi, Bryssinckx, Welburn, and Moriyon, 2014). For example, peoples' decision to attend or ignore physical or psychological changes, their interpretation and evaluation of the change and their ways of responding to the symptoms of a disease are influenced by culture (Fenichel, 2013; Fenichel et al., 2011; Fogel, 1994). Hence public health measures have to consider the cultural background, i.e., the social agreements and assumptions and must be located at the community level to enhance in-depth understanding of the individual context, participation, and appropriateness of measures (Narrod, Zinsstag, and Tiongco, 2012; Nascimento and de Oliveira, 2014; O'Brien, Lahue, Caro, and Davidson, 2007). However, there is a lack of necessary qualitative research within public health and measures often rely on assumptions of culture and cultural practices (Casamassimo, Thikkurissy, Edelstein, and Maiorini, 2009; Castro, Wilson, and Bloom, 2017).

This can lead to public health responses being ineffective or even harmful (Abegunde and Stanciole, 2008; Abramowitz, Lacau Saint Guily, Moyal-Barracco, Bergeron, Borne, Dahlab, and Bénard, 2018). While epidemic outbreaks such as HIV/AIDS led to an increase in cultural awareness the response to recent epidemics show that there is still a lot to learn (Acemoglu and Johnson, 2007; Adda, 2016; Alloul, Sauriol, Kennedy, Laurier, Tessier, Novosel, and Contandriopoulos, 1998). This is particularly true with reference to Western-educated clinicians who are sometimes called to respond to emerging pandemics in the developing world (Amuna and Zotor, 2008; Aral, Holmes, Padian, and Cates, 1996; Arbabi, Nezami, Hooshyar, and Delavari, 2018). Importing their own cultural practices and prejudices can render their responses irrelevant and therefore ineffective (Armelagos, Brown, and Turner, 2005; Arokiasamy and Krishnan, 1994; Arora, 2001, 2005; Arredondo and Zúñiga, 2004). As Figure 2.3 shows, there is no shortage of urgent research and development projects related to disease epidemics.

DISEASE	DESCRIPTION	BIOMEDICAL COUNTERMEASURES
Crimean-Congo hemorrhagic fever (CCHF)	Hemorrhagic fever caused by virus transmitted through ticks and livestock, with case-fatality rate of up to 40%. Human-to-human transmission is possible.	No vaccine available; ribavirin (antiviral) provides some treatment benefit.
Ebola virus disease	Hemorrhagic fever caused by virus transmitted by wild animals, with case-fatality rate of up to 90%. Human-to-human transmission is possible.	Experimental vaccine available
Marburg virus disease	Hemorrhagic fever caused by virus transmitted by fruit bats, with case-fatality rate of up to 88%. Human-to-human transmission is possible.	No vaccine available
Lassa fever	Hemorrhagic fever caused by virus transmitted through contact with rodent urine or feces, with case-fatality rate of 15% in severe cases. Human-to-human transmission is possible.	No vaccine available Vaccine development funded by CEPI
Middle East respiratory syndrome coronavirus (MERS-CoV)	Respiratory disease caused by a coronavirus transmitted by camels and humans, with case-fatality rate of 35%.	No vaccine available Vaccine development funded by CEPI
Severe acute respiratory syndrome (SARS)	Respiratory disease caused by a coronavirus transmitted from human to human and from animals (possibly bats), with a case-fatality rate of 10%.	No vaccine available
Nipah and henipaviral diseases	Disease caused by a virus transmitted by fruit bats, pigs, and humans; can manifest as an acute respiratory syndrome or encephalitis. Case-fatality rate can reach 100%.	Vaccine development funded by CEPI
Rift Valley fever (RVF)	Disease caused by a virus transmitted by contact with the blood or organs of infected animals, or by mosquitos. Up to 50% case-fatality rate in patients with hemorrhagic fever. No human-to-human transmission has been reported.	Experimental, unlicensed vaccine available
Zika	Disease caused by a flavivirus transmitted by mosquitoes. Can result in microcephaly in infants born to infected mothers and in Guillain-Barré syndrome. Human-to-human transmission is possible.	No vaccine available
Disease X (pathogens currently unknown to cause human disease)	N/A	CEPI is funding the development of institutional and technical platforms that allow for rapid R&D in response to outbreaks of pathogens for which no vaccine exists.

Figure 2.3. Diseases requirement research and development attention in 2018.

Source: IMF.

However, the cultural aspects are not yet fully investigated (Arredondo and Zúñiga, 2006; Backer, van Roermund, Fischer, van Asseldonk, and Bergevoet, 2015; Bartsch, Hotez, Hertenstein, Diemert, Zapf, Bottazzi, and Lee, 2016).

Culture has been shown to affect "the various ways that HIV/AIDS has impacted on the African population as a case in point (Bausch and Schwarz, 2014; Bausch et al., 2001; Benner, Carabin, Sánchez-Serrano, Budke, and Carmena, 2010). This is partially because sexuality is socially constructed phenomenon and culture and culturally embedded beliefs and values can influence sexual norms, definition of sexual orientation and stigmatization of certain groups (Bergevoet, Van Schaik, Veling, Backus, and Franken, 2009; Binder, 1988; Bolos, Bacarea, and Marusteri, 2011). For instance, social stigma linked to purchasing condoms, male dominance or cultural embedded views on fertility can affect HIV prevention and lead to a high burden of HIV being placed on women (Bonds, Keenan, Rohani, and Sachs, 2010; Boni, Galvani, Wickelgren, and Malani, 2013; Bonovas and Nikolopoulos, 2012). Public health measures to stop the HIV/AIDS epidemic did not consider such cultural aspects at first (Borghol, Suderman, McArdle, Racine, Hallett, Pembrey, and Szyf, 2012; Brandes, 2008; Brown, Lipscomb, and Snyder, 2001). However, international development agencies quickly realized that a medical approach alone is not sufficient to tackle a multifaceted issue as HIV/AIDS and similar pandemics (Buckley, 1984; Budke, Jiamin, Qian, and Torgerson, 2005; Bundy, Arámbulo III, and Grey, 1983; Buzby and Roberts, 2009). Yet, the motivation for this shift was mainly driven by the need for more effective interventions (Bwire, Munier, Ouedraogo, Heyerdahl, Komakech, Kagirita, and Makumbi, 2017; Canali, Aragrande, Angheben, Capelli, Drigo, Gobbi, and Cassini, 2020). This corresponds with the common deficit orientated understanding of culture in public health research (Casamassimo, Thikkurissy, Edelstein, and Maiorini, 2009; Castro, Wilson, and Bloom, 2017).

In recent years, the world has witnessed a number of epidemic outbreaks with devastating effects (Chen, Li, Hsieh, Chang, Lee, Lee, and Ko, 2012; Conover, Pitt, Kessler, DuBow, and Sanborn, 1995; Crump, Murdoch, and Baker, 2001). While outbreaks are inevitable, their impact can be mitigated (Daily, and Ehrlich, 1996; Deogaonkar, Hutubessy, Van Der Putten, Evers, and Jit, 2012; Dorn, 1992; Ducrotoy, Bertu, Ocholi, Gusi, Bryssinckx, Welburn, and Moriyon, 2014). Effective management of such events calls for better approaches encompassing all the different aspects that can influence the outcome, including the cultural aspect (Eaton and Groopman, 2013;

Eckelman, Sherman, and MacNeill, 2018; Egger, 2011; Elbe, 2007; Ernst and Hay, 1994). Communities' response to outbreaks and their willingness to embrace the interventions devised and implemented by international experts in order to mitigate the effects of an outbreak can greatly influence the outcome (Espinoza, Terashima, Herrera-Velit, and Marcos, 2010; Ezzati, Vander Hoorn, Lawes, Leach, James, Lopez, and Murray, 2005). There have been considerable challenges in managing outbreaks in some parts of Africa due to the strong influence of traditional beliefs with regard to the response to the outbreaks and to the measures instituted to counter them (Fenichel, 2013; Fenichel et al., 2011; Fogel, 1994). The outbreak of the Zika virus, similarly, presented unanticipated healthcare challenges (Foxman, 2002; Garner, Whan, Gard, and Phillips, 2001; Gayle and Hill, 2001; Gottstein, Pozio, and Nöckler, 2009). The case of the Ebola pandemic in West Africa can help develop a deeper insight into the issue of pandemics and the cultural response observed and its effect on the outcome of the event (Hart and Halden, 2020; Häsler, Howe, and Stärk, 2011; Henschke, Kamper, and Maher, 2015; Hochberg, 1992).

Given the challenges faced with ongoing efforts to contain the spread of Ebola that arose as a result of incompatibilities between some religious and cultural practices and prescribed scientific methods, it is appropriate to explore ways in which traditional and religious structures can be effectively utilized in combatting the spread of Ebola (Howe, Häsler, and Stärk, 2013; Howe et al., 2012). Dealing with cultural and religious issues negatively will affect Ebola transmission prevention programs and will require flexibility and adaptability from governments, health officials, and the people in affected communities (Jenkins, Baingana, Ahmad, McDaid, and Atun, 2011; Johnson, Alvarez-Pasquin, Bijl, Franco, Gaillat, Clara, and Weinke, 2015). A consideration of traditional and religious practices is critical to our understanding of transmission dynamics and subsequent control of highly infectious diseases (Kim and Goldie, 2008; Klein, Laxminarayan, Smith, and Gilligan, 2007; Klepac, Laxminarayan, and Grenfell, 2011). Researchers have identified notable religious and traditional practices in West Africa that potentially contribute to the spread of Ebola and exacerbate the current outbreak to state an example (Krieger, 2001a, b; Lemma, 1969; Liu, Maniadakis, Gray, and Rayner, 2002; López, Torné, Franco, San-Martin, Viayna, Barrull, and Perulero, 2018). Some of the proposed strategies call for deliberate targeting of leaders of traditional and religious institutions in community-directed programs for preventive measures (Markos and Abdela, 2016; Martin and Shepherd, 2009; McGuinness, McGlynn,

Johnson, MacIntyre, Batty, Burns, and McGinty, 2012). As custodians of the day-to-day cultural values, traditional, and religious leaders command more respect and authority in their communities than unfamiliar yet trained health personnel, who can be easily be viewed as having duplicitous agendas (Moné, Ibikounlé, Massougbodji, and Mouahid, 2010; Morand, 2004; Moro, Budke, Schantz, Vasquez, Santivanez, and Villavicencio, 2011).

The Ebola virus epidemic in West Africa has had a large effect on the culture of most of the West African countries (Narrod, Zinsstag, and Tiongco, 2012; Nascimento and de Oliveira, 2014; O'Brien, Lahue, Caro, and Davidson, 2007). In most instances, the effect is a rather negative one as it has disrupted many Africans' traditional norms and practices (Oleś, Gudowska-Nowak, and Kleczkowski, 2012; Otte, Nugent, and McLeod, 2004; Ozawa, Portnoy, Getaneh, Clark, Knoll, Bishai, and Patwardhan, 2016). For instance, many West African communities rely on traditional healers and witch doctors, who use herbal remedies, massage, chant, and witchcraft to cure just about any ailment (Ozmen, Kurşun, and Ozcelik, 2005; Paarlberg, Hillberg, Lee, and Mathews, 2008; Paisley, Vraa-Andersen, Dybkjaer, Møller, Christensen, Mousing, and Agger, 1993). Therefore, it is difficult for West Africans to adapt to foreign medical practices (Pal, Kerorsa, Marami, and Kandi, 2020; Paterson, Otte, Slingenbergh, Wint, and Rogers, 2000; Pearce and Merletti, 2006). Specifically, West African resistance to Western medicine is prominent in the region, which calls for severe distrust of Western and modern medical personnel and practices (Peckham, 2013; Perrings et al., 2002, 2014). Similarly, some African cultures have a traditional solidarity of standing by the sick, which is contrary to the safe care of an Ebola patient (Perry and Randolph, 1999; Philipson, 2000; Philipson and Posner, 1996; Pongchaiyakul, Songpattanasilp, and Taechakraichana, 2008). This tradition is known as "standing by the ill" in order to show one's respect and honor to the patient (Poundstone, Strathdee, and Celentano, 2004; Pritchett, Thilmany, and Johnson, 2005; Pugliatti, Beghi, Forsgren, Ekman, and Sobocki, 2007). According to the Wesley Medical Center, these sorts of traditional norms can be dangerous to those not infected with the virus as it increases their chances of coming in contact with their family member's bodily fluids (Purevdawa, Moon, Baigalmaa, Davaajav, Smith, and Vermund, 1997; Ramesh, Malla, Raju, Sehgal, Ganguly, Mahajan, and Dilawari, 1990). In Liberia, Ebola has wiped out entire families, leaving perhaps one survivor to recount stories of how they simply could not be hands-off while their loved ones were sick in bed, because of their culture of touch, hold, hug, and kiss (Raut, 2004; Rehm, Mathers, Popova,

Thavorncharoensap, Teerawattananon, and Patra, 2009; Rich and Perry, 2011). Some communities traditionally use folklore and mythical literature, which is often passed on verbally from one generation to the next to explain the interrelationships of all things that exist (Rogers, Carolin, Vaught, and Compton, 2011; Ronohardjo and Rastiko, 1982; Sachs, 2001; Sachs and Malaney, 2002). However, the folklore and songs are not only of traditional or ancient historical origins, but are often about current events that have affected the community (Saleha, 1991; Sibert, Rigaud, Delavierre, and Labat, 2010; Skrepnek and Skrepnek, 2004; Sloane, 2009; Sockett, 1993). Additionally, folklore, and music will often take opposing sides of any story (St George, 1986; Steben and Duarte-Franco, 2007; Stehr-Green and Schantz, 1987; Stuckler, 2008; Stuckler and Siegel, 2011). Thus early in the Ebola epidemic, the song "White Ebola" was released by a diaspora-based group and centers on the general distrust of "outsiders" who may be intentionally infecting people (Suhrcke, Stuckler, Suk, Desai, Senek, McKee, and Rechel, 2011; Šumilo, Bormane, Asokliene, Vasilenko, Golovljova, Avsic-Zupanc, and Randolph, 2008). This initial misinformation increased the general distrust in foreigners, and the idea that Ebola was not in Africa before their arrival led to attacks on many health workers, as well as blockages of aid convoys blocked from checking remote areas (Tapia, 2003; Torgerson and Dowling, 2001; Torgerson, Carmona, and Bonifacino, 2000; Uddin Khan, Atanasova, Krueger, Ramirez, and Gray, 2013).

The Ebola epidemic of 2014 has forced West Africans to face numerous difficulties on a daily basis regarding their traditional norms and practices (Uusküla, Müürsepp, Kawai, Raag, Jürisson, and Pillsbury, 2013; Vanni, Karnon, Madan, White, Edmunds, Foss, and Legood, 2011). In essence, their traditions have been severely disrupted due to the Ebola virus (Weycker, Edelsberg, Oster, and Tino, 2005; Wu, Perrings, Kinzig, Collins, Minteer, and Daszak, 2017; Yach, Stuckler, and Brownell, 2006). For instance, West Africans have had the tendency to remain close to their sick family members to nurse them during illness for centuries (Yi-Xin and Manderson, 2005; Zadoks, 2008; Zhan, Li, Wang, Sun, Geng, Xiong, and de Hoog, 2015; Zhang, Song, Cai, and Zhou, 2008). Unfortunately for West African communities, many have been encouraged to keep their distance from their infected family members as potential contact could be fatal (Casamassimo, Thikkurissy, Edelstein, and Maiorini, 2009; Castro, Wilson, and Bloom, 2017). The next section considers the lifestyle aspects of disease pandemics.

2.4. LIFESTYLE ASPECTS OF DISEASE EPIDEMICS

There are some disease epidemics that are caused or sustained by lifestyle aspects such as diet, rest, and exercise (Narrod, Zinsstag, and Tiongco, 2012; Nascimento and de Oliveira, 2014; O'Brien, Lahue, Caro, and Davidson, 2007). Lifestyle diseases are defined as diseases linked with the way people live their life. These are non-communicable diseases (Fenichel, 2013; Fenichel et al., 2011; Fogel, 1994). This is commonly caused by lack of physical activity, unhealthy eating, alcohol, drugs, and smoking. Diseases that mostly have an effect on our lifestyle are heart disease, stroke, obesity, and type II diabetes (Daily, and Ehrlich, 1996; Deogaonkar, Hutubessy, Van Der Putten, Evers, and Jit, 2012; Dorn, 1992; Ducrotoy, Bertu, Ocholi, Gusi, Bryssinckx, Welburn, and Moriyon, 2014). The diseases that appear to increase in frequency as countries become more industrialized and people live longer can include Alzheimer's disease, arthritis, atherosclerosis, asthma, cancer, chronic liver disease or cirrhosis, chronic obstructive pulmonary disease (COPD), colitis, irritable bowel syndrome, type 2 diabetes, heart disease, hypertension, metabolic syndrome, chronic kidney failure, osteoporosis, PCOD, stroke, depression, obesity, and vascular dementia (Peckham, 2013; Perrings et al., 2002, 2014). Just like other communicable diseases (see Figure 2.4 for the example of Ebola impacting on agriculture); lifestyle disease may impact on economic activity and human participation due to infirmities and fatalities.

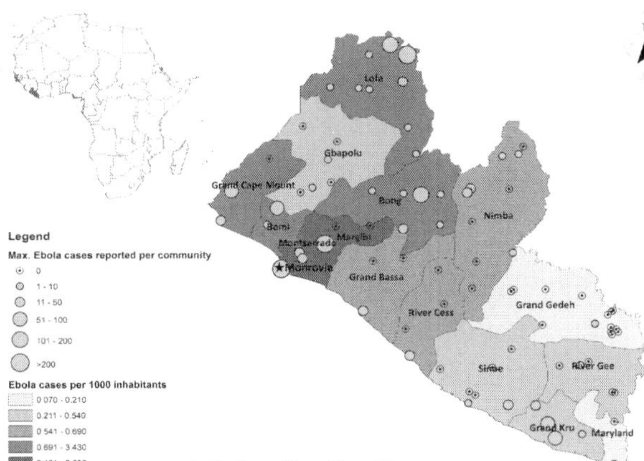

Figure 2.4. Impact of Ebola pandemic on agricultural activities.

Source: PLoS.

Some commenters maintain a distinction between diseases of longevity and diseases of civilization or diseases of affluence (Saleha, 1991; Sibert, Rigaud, Delavierre, and Labat, 2010; Skrepnek and Skrepnek, 2004; Sloane, 2009; Sockett, 1993). Certain diseases, such as diabetes, dental caries, and asthma, appear at greater rates in young populations living in the "western" way (Tapia, 2003; Torgerson and Dowling, 2001; Torgerson, Carmona, and Bonifacino, 2000; Uddin Khan, Atanasova, Krueger, Ramirez, and Gray, 2013). Hence, their increased incidence is not related to age, so the terms cannot accurately be used interchangeably for all diseases (Borghol, Suderman, McArdle, Racine, Hallett, Pembrey, and Szyf, 2012; Brandes, 2008; Brown, Lipscomb, and Snyder, 2001). Diet and lifestyle are major factors thought to influence susceptibility to many diseases (Purevdawa, Moon, Baigalmaa, Davaajav, Smith, and Vermund, 1997; Ramesh, Malla, Raju, Sehgal, Ganguly, Mahajan, and Dilawari, 1990). Drug abuse, tobacco smoking, and alcohol drinking, as well as a lack of or excessive exercise may also increase the risk of developing certain diseases, especially later in life (Bausch and Schwarz, 2014; Bausch et al., 2001; Benner, Carabin, Sánchez-Serrano, Budke, and Carmena, 2010). In many Western countries, people began to consume more meat, dairy products, vegetable oils, tobacco, sugary foods, sugary beverages, and alcoholic beverages during the latter half of the 20th century (Rogers, Carolin, Vaught, and Compton, 2011; Ronohardjo and Rastiko, 1982; Sachs, 2001; Sachs and Malaney, 2002). People also developed sedentary lifestyles and greater rates of obesity (Oleś, Gudowska-Nowak, and Kleczkowski, 2012; Otte, Nugent, and McLeod, 2004; Ozawa, Portnoy, Getaneh, Clark, Knoll, Bishai, and Patwardhan, 2016).

Rates of colorectal cancer, breast cancer, prostate cancer, endometrial cancer and lung cancer started increasing noticeably after this dietary change (Eaton and Groopman, 2013; Eckelman, Sherman, and MacNeill, 2018; Egger, 2011; Elbe, 2007; Ernst and Hay, 1994). People in developing countries, whose diets still depended largely on low-sugar starchy foods with little meat or fat were seen to have lower rates of these cancers (Moné, Ibikounlé, Massougbodji, and Mouahid, 2010; Morand, 2004; Moro, Budke, Schantz, Vasquez, Santivanez, and Villavicencio, 2011). Causes are not just from smoking and alcohol abuse (Foxman, 2002; Garner, Whan, Gard, and Phillips, 2001; Gayle and Hill, 2001; Gottstein, Pozio, and Nöckler, 2009). Adults can develop lifestyle diseases through behavioral factors that impact on them (Markos and Abdela, 2016; Martin and Shepherd, 2009; McGuinness, McGlynn, Johnson, MacIntyre, Batty, Burns, and McGinty, 2012). These can be unemployment, unsafe living, poor social environment, working conditions, stress, and home life can change a person's lifestyle to increase their risk of developing one of these diseases (Hart and Halden, 2020; Häsler, Howe, and Stärk, 2011; Henschke, Kamper, and Maher, 2015; Hochberg, 1992). There is a lot of statistical evidence of an increase in these lifestyle diseases among developed nations such as Australia (Raut, 2004; Rehm, Mathers, Popova, Thavorncharoensap, Teerawattananon, and Patra, 2009; Rich and Perry, 2011). Between 1995 and 2005, 813,000 Australians were hospitalized due to alcohol (Howe, Häsler, and Stärk, 2013; Howe et al., 2012). In 2014, about 11.2 million Australians were deemed to be overweight or obese (Arredondo and Zúñiga, 2006; Backer, van Roermund, Fischer, van Asseldonk, and Bergevoet, 2015; Bartsch, Hotez, Hertenstein, Diemert, Zapf, Bottazzi, and Lee, 2016).

In 1900, the top three causes of death in the United States were pneumonia or influenza, tuberculosis, and diarrhea or enteritis (Bergevoet, Van Schaik, Veling, Backus, and Franken, 2009; Binder, 1988; Bolos, Bacarea, and Marusteri, 2011). Communicable diseases accounted for about 60% of all deaths (Suhrcke, Stuckler, Suk, Desai, Senek, McKee, and Rechel, 2011; Šumilo, Bormane, Asokliene, Vasilenko, Golovljova, Avsic-Zupanc, and Randolph, 2008). In 1900, heart disease and cancer were ranked number 4 and 8 respectively (Poundstone, Strathdee, and Celentano, 2004; Pritchett, Thilmany, and Johnson, 2005; Pugliatti, Beghi, Forsgren, Ekman, and Sobocki, 2007). Since the 1940s, the majority of deaths in the United States have resulted from heart disease, cancer, and other degenerative diseases (Armelagos, Brown, and Turner, 2005; Arokiasamy and Krishnan, 1994; Arora, 2001, 2005; Arredondo and Zúñiga, 2004). By the late 1990s, degenerative diseases accounted for more than 60% of all deaths (Krieger, 2001a, b; Lemma, 1969; Liu, Maniadakis, Gray, and Rayner, 2002; López, Torné, Franco, San-Martin, Viayna, Barrull, and Perulero, 2018). Lifestyle diseases have their onset later in an individual's life (Amuna and Zotor, 2008; Aral, Holmes, Padian, and Cates, 1996; Arbabi, Nezami, Hooshyar, and Delavari, 2018). They appear to increase in frequency as countries become more industrialized and people live longer (Acemoglu and Johnson, 2007; Adda, 2016; Alloul, Sauriol, Kennedy, Laurier, Tessier, Novosel, and Contandriopoulos, 1998). This suggests that the life expectancy at birth of 49.24 years in 1900 was too short for degenerative diseases to occur, compared to a life expectancy at birth of 77.8 years in 2004 (St George, 1986; Steben and Duarte-Franco, 2007; Stehr-Green and Schantz, 1987; Stuckler, 2008; Stuckler and Siegel, 2011). Moreover, survivorship to the age of 50 was 58.5% in 1900, and 93.7% in 2007 (Uusküla, Müürsepp,

Kawai, Raag, Jürisson, and Pillsbury, 2013; Vanni, Karnon, Madan, White, Edmunds, Foss, and Legood, 2011).

Prevention is remedies or activities that aim to reduce the likelihood of a disease or disorder affecting people (Perry and Randolph, 1999; Philipson, 2000; Philipson and Posner, 1996; Pongchaiyakul, Songpattanasilp, and Taechakraichana, 2008). Lifestyle diseases are preventable for children if parents set them on the correct path, as early life decisions and influences can impact people later on in life (Weycker, Edelsberg, Oster, and Tino, 2005; Wu, Perrings, Kinzig, Collins, Minteer, and Daszak, 2017; Yach, Stuckler, and Brownell, 2006). Lifestyle diseases can be prevented through reduction in smoking of tobacco (Chen, Li, Hsieh, Chang, Lee, Lee, and Ko, 2012; Conover, Pitt, Kessler, DuBow, and Sanborn, 1995; Crump, Murdoch, and Baker, 2001). Some governments have started this by introducing plain packaging for all tobacco products and increasing the prices of tobacco production (Kim and Goldie, 2008; Klein, Laxminarayan, Smith, and Gilligan, 2007; Klepac, Laxminarayan, and Grenfell, 2011). Being overweight and morbid obesity can be prevented through a well-balanced lifestyle through healthy eating and exercise (Abegunde and Stanciole, 2008; Abramowitz, Lacau Saint Guily, Moyal-Barracco, Bergeron, Borne, Dahlab, and Bénard, 2018). In addition, animal studies have suggested that early life exercise can reduce the risk of developing metabolic diseases in adulthood (Jenkins, Baingana, Ahmad, McDaid, and Atun, 2011; Johnson, Alvarez-Pasquin, Bijl, Franco, Gaillat, Clara, and Weinke, 2015). This chapter will look at disease epidemics that occur as a consequence of bio weaponry.

2.5. BIO-WEAPONRY AND DISEASE EPIDEMICS

Setting aside, the onset of conspiracy theories in the age of online chatrooms; bio weaponry and its use in biowarfare can represent significant dangers to the human population (Pal, Kerorsa, Marami, and Kandi, 2020; Paterson, Otte, Slingenbergh, Wint, and Rogers, 2000; Pearce and Merletti, 2006). Biological warfare, also known as germ warfare, is the use of biological toxins or infectious agents such as bacteria, viruses, insects, and fungi with the intent to kill or incapacitate humans, animals or plants as an act of war (Yi-Xin and Manderson, 2005; Zadoks, 2008; Zhan, Li, Wang, Sun, Geng, Xiong, and de Hoog, 2015; Zhang, Song, Cai, and Zhou, 2008). Biological weapons (often termed "bio-weapons," "biological threat agents," or "bio-agents") are living organisms or replicating entities or viruses, which are not universally considered "alive" (Bwire, Munier, Ouedraogo, Heyerdahl, Komakech, Kagirita, and Makumbi, 2017; Canali, Aragrande, Angheben, Capelli, Drigo, Gobbi, and Cassini, 2020). Entomological (insect) warfare is a subtype of biowarfare (Buckley, 1984; Budke, Jiamin, Qian, and Torgerson, 2005; Bundy, Arámbulo III, and Grey, 1983; Buzby and Roberts, 2009). As Figure 2.5, there is significant potential for developing new and deadly bio weaponry in the future.

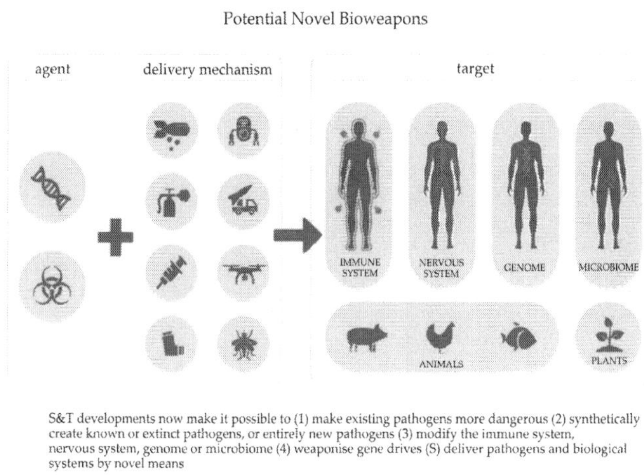

Figure 2.5. Potential bioweapons.

Source: Dr. Fillippa Lentzos.

Biological warfare is distinct from nuclear warfare, chemical warfare and radiological warfare, which together with biological warfare make up the military initialism for nuclear, biological, radiological, and chemical warfare using weapons of mass destruction (Espinoza, Terashima, Herrera-Velit, and Marcos, 2010; Ezzati, Vander Hoorn, Lawes, Leach, James, Lopez, and Murray, 2005). None of these are considered conventional weapons, which are deployed primarily for their explosive, kinetic, or incendiary potential (Bonds, Keenan, Rohani, and Sachs, 2010; Boni, Galvani, Wickelgren, and Malani, 2013; Bonovas and Nikolopoulos, 2012). Biological weapons may be employed in various ways to gain a strategic or tactical advantage over the enemy, either by threats or by actual deployments (Ozmen, Kurşun, and Ozcelik, 2005; Paarlberg, Hillberg, Lee, and Mathews, 2008; Paisley, Vraa-Andersen, Dybkjaer, Møller, Christensen, Mousing, and Agger, 1993). Like some chemical weapons, biological weapons may also be useful as area denial weapons. These agents may be lethal or non-lethal, and may be targeted against a single individual, a group of people, or even an entire population (Casamassimo, Thikkurissy, Edelstein, and Maiorini, 2009; Castro, Wilson, and Bloom, 2017). They may be developed, acquired, stockpiled or deployed by nation-states or by non-national groups (Poundstone, Strathdee, and Celentano, 2004; Pritchett, Thilmany, and Johnson, 2005; Pugliatti, Beghi, Forsgren, Ekman, and Sobocki, 2007). In the latter case, or if a nation-state uses it clandestinely, it may also be considered bioterrorism (St George, 1986; Steben and Duarte-Franco, 2007; Stehr-Green and Schantz, 1987; Stuckler, 2008; Stuckler and Siegel, 2011).

Biological warfare and chemical warfare overlap to a certain extent, as the use of toxins produced by some living organisms is considered under the provisions of both the Biological Weapons Convention and the Chemical Weapons Convention (Kim and Goldie, 2008; Klein, Laxminarayan, Smith, and Gilligan, 2007; Klepac, Laxminarayan, and Grenfell, 2011). Toxins and psychochemical weapons are often referred to as mid-spectrum agents (Bonds, Keenan, Rohani, and Sachs, 2010; Boni, Galvani, Wickelgren, and Malani, 2013; Bonovas and Nikolopoulos, 2012). Unlike bioweapons, these mid-spectrum agents do not reproduce in their host and are typically characterized by shorter incubation periods (Oleś, Gudowska-Nowak, and Kleczkowski, 2012; Otte, Nugent, and McLeod, 2004; Ozawa, Portnoy, Getaneh, Clark, Knoll, Bishai, and Patwardhan, 2016). The use of biological weapons is prohibited under customary international humanitarian law, as well as a variety of international treaties (Armelagos, Brown, and Turner, 2005; Arokiasamy and Krishnan, 1994; Arora, 2001, 2005; Arredondo and Zúñiga, 2004). The use of biological agents in armed conflict is a war crime (Bwire, Munier, Ouedraogo, Heyerdahl, Komakech, Kagirita, and Makumbi, 2017; Canali, Aragrande, Angheben, Capelli, Drigo, Gobbi, and Cassini, 2020). Offensive biological warfare, including mass production, stockpiling, and use of biological weapons, was outlawed by 1972 under the Biological Weapons Convention (Borghol, Suderman, McArdle, Racine, Hallett, Pembrey, and Szyf, 2012; Brandes, 2008; Brown, Lipscomb, and Snyder, 2001). The rationale behind this treaty (ratified or acceded to by 170 countries by April 2013) is to prevent a biological attack which could conceivably result in large numbers of civilian casualties and cause severe disruption to be economic and societal infrastructure (Peckham, 2013; Perrings et al., 2002, 2014). Many countries, including signatories of the Biological Weapons Convention, currently pursue research into the defense or protection against biowarfare, which is not prohibited by the convention

(Amuna and Zotor, 2008; Aral, Holmes, Padian, and Cates, 1996; Arbabi, Nezami, Hooshyar, and Delavari, 2018).

A nation or group that can pose a credible threat of mass casualty has the ability to alter the terms under which other nations or groups interact with it (Acemoglu and Johnson, 2007; Adda, 2016; Alloul, Sauriol, Kennedy, Laurier, Tessier, Novosel, and Contandriopoulos, 1998). When indexed to weapon mass and cost of development and storage, biological weapons possess destructive potential and loss of life far in excess of nuclear, chemical, or conventional weapons (Eaton and Groopman, 2013; Eckelman, Sherman, and MacNeill, 2018; Egger, 2011; Elbe, 2007; Ernst and Hay, 1994). Accordingly, biological agents are potentially useful as strategic deterrents, in addition to their utility as offensive weapons on the battlefield (Espinoza, Terashima, Herrera-Velit, and Marcos, 2010; Ezzati, Vander Hoorn, Lawes, Leach, James, Lopez, and Murray, 2005). As a tactical weapon for military use, a significant problem with a bio weaponry attack is that it would take days to be effective, and therefore might not immediately stop an opposing force (Markos and Abdela, 2016; Martin and Shepherd, 2009; McGuinness, McGlynn, Johnson, MacIntyre, Batty, Burns, and McGinty, 2012).

Some biological agents (smallpox, pneumonic plague) have the capability of person-to-person transmission via aerosolized respiratory droplets (Suhrcke, Stuckler, Suk, Desai, Senek, McKee, and Rechel, 2011; Šumilo, Bormane, Asokliene, Vasilenko, Golovljova, Avsic-Zupanc, and Randolph, 2008). This feature can be undesirable, as the agents may be transmitted by this mechanism to unintended populations, including neutral or even friendly forces (Bergevoet, Van Schaik, Veling, Backus, and Franken, 2009; Binder, 1988; Bolos, Bacarea, and Marusteri, 2011). Worse still, such a weapon could "escape" the laboratory where it was developed, even if there was no intent to use it (Tapia, 2003; Torgerson and Dowling, 2001; Torgerson, Carmona, and Bonifacino, 2000; Uddin Khan, Atanasova, Krueger, Ramirez, and Gray, 2013). For example, the agent could be spread by infecting a researcher who then transmits it to the outside world before realizing that they were infected (Moné, Ibikounlé, Massougbodji, and Mouahid, 2010; Morand, 2004; Moro, Budke, Schantz, Vasquez, Santivanez, and Villavicencio, 2011). Several cases are known of researchers becoming infected and dying of Ebola, while they had been working within the lab (Uusküla, Müürsepp, Kawai, Raag, Jürisson, and Pillsbury, 2013; Vanni, Karnon, Madan, White, Edmunds, Foss, and Legood, 2011). However, nobody else was infected in those cases (Raut, 2004; Rehm, Mathers, Popova, Thavorncharoensap, Teerawattananon, and Patra, 2009; Rich and

Perry, 2011). While there is no evidence that their work was directed towards bio weaponry, it demonstrates the potential for accidental infection even of careful researchers fully aware of the dangers (Foxman, 2002; Garner, Whan, Gard, and Phillips, 2001; Gayle and Hill, 2001; Gottstein, Pozio, and Nöckler, 2009). While containment of bio weaponry is less of a concern for certain criminal or terrorist organizations, it remains a significant concern for the military and civilian populations of virtually all nations (Howe, Häsler, and Stärk, 2013; Howe et al., 2012).

Rudimentary forms of biological warfare have been practiced since antiquity (Weycker, Edelsberg, Oster, and Tino, 2005; Wu, Perrings, Kinzig, Collins, Minteer, and Daszak, 2017; Yach, Stuckler, and Brownell, 2006). The earliest documented incident of the intention to use biological weapons is recorded in Hittite texts of 1500–1200; BC (Daily, and Ehrlich, 1996; Deogaonkar, Hutubessy, Van Der Putten, Evers, and Jit, 2012; Dorn, 1992; Ducrotoy, Bertu, Ocholi, Gusi, Bryssinckx, Welburn, and Moriyon, 2014). Here, the victims of tularemia were driven into enemy lands, causing an epidemic (Chen, Li, Hsieh, Chang, Lee, Lee, and Ko, 2012; Conover, Pitt, Kessler, DuBow, and Sanborn, 1995; Crump, Murdoch, and Baker, 2001). Although the Assyrians knew of ergot, a parasitic fungus of rye which produces ergotism when ingested, there is no evidence that they poisoned enemy wells with the fungus, as has been claimed (Arredondo and Zúñiga, 2006; Backer, van Roermund, Fischer, van Asseldonk, and Bergevoet, 2015; Bartsch, Hotez, Hertenstein, Diemert, Zapf, Bottazzi, and Lee, 2016). Scythian archers dipped their arrows and Roman soldiers their swords into excrements and cadavers so that victims were commonly infected by tetanus as a result (Rogers, Carolin, Vaught, and Compton, 2011; Ronohardjo and Rastiko, 1982; Sachs, 2001; Sachs and Malaney, 2002).

There are other examples of aspects or even early attempts at the use of bio weaponry, even if that use was not as deadly as the modern usage (Yi-Xin and Manderson, 2005; Zadoks, 2008; Zhan, Li, Wang, Sun, Geng, Xiong, and de Hoog, 2015; Zhang, Song, Cai, and Zhou, 2008). For example, in 1346 the bodies of Mongol warriors of the Golden Horde who had died of plague were thrown over the walls of the besieged Crimean city of Kaffa (Perry and Randolph, 1999; Philipson, 2000; Philipson and Posner, 1996; Pongchaiyakul, Songpattanasilp, and Taechakraichana, 2008). Specialists disagree about whether this operation was responsible for the spread of the Black Death into Europe, Near East, and North Africa (Abegunde and Stanciole, 2008; Abramowitz, Lacau Saint Guily, Moyal-Barracco, Bergeron, Borne, Dahlab, and Bénard, 2018). This is the pandemic that resulted in the deaths of approximately 25 million Europeans (Fenichel, 2013; Fenichel et al., 2011; Fogel, 1994). Biological weaponry were extensively used in many parts of Africa from the 16th century AD, most of the time in the form of poisoned arrows, or powder spread on the war front as well as poisoning of horses and water supply of the enemy forces (Saleha, 1991; Sibert, Rigaud, Delavierre, and Labat, 2010; Skrepnek and Skrepnek, 2004; Sloane, 2009; Sockett, 1993). In Borgu for example, there were specific mixtures to kill, hypnotize, make the enemy bold, and to act as an antidote against the poison of the enemy as well (Bausch and Schwarz, 2014; Bausch et al., 2001; Benner, Carabin, Sánchez-Serrano, Budke, and Carmena, 2010).

More recently, there have been disturbing incidents of bio weaponry being deployed (Hart and Halden, 2020; Häsler, Howe, and Stärk, 2011; Henschke, Kamper, and Maher, 2015; Hochberg, 1992). The British Army, for example, attempted use of smallpox against Native Americans during the Siege of Fort Pitt in June 1763 (Ozmen, Kurşun, and Ozcelik, 2005; Paarlberg, Hillberg, Lee, and Mathews, 2008; Paisley, Vraa-Andersen, Dybkjaer, Møller, Christensen, Mousing, and Agger, 1993). A reported outbreak that began the spring before left as many as 100 Native Americans dead in Ohio Country from 1763 to 1764 (Buckley, 1984; Budke, Jiamin, Qian, and Torgerson, 2005; Bundy, Arámbulo III, and Grey, 1983; Buzby and Roberts, 2009). It is not clear, however, whether the smallpox was a result of the Fort Pitt incident or the virus was already present among the Delaware people as outbreaks happened on their own every dozen or so years (Pal, Kerorsa, Marami, and Kandi, 2020; Paterson, Otte, Slingenbergh, Wint, and Rogers, 2000; Pearce and Merletti, 2006). Indeed, the delegates were met again later and seemingly had not contracted smallpox (Narrod, Zinsstag, and Tiongco, 2012; Nascimento and de Oliveira, 2014; O'Brien, Lahue, Caro, and Davidson, 2007). It is likely that the British Marines used smallpox in New South Wales, Australia, in 1789. Dr. Seth Carus (2015) states: "*Ultimately, we have a strong circumstantial case supporting the theory that someone deliberately introduced smallpox in the Aboriginal population.*"

By 1900 the germ theory and advances in bacteriology brought a new level of sophistication to the techniques for possible use of bio-agents in war (Krieger, 2001a, b; Lemma, 1969; Liu, Maniadakis, Gray, and Rayner, 2002; López, Torné, Franco, San-Martin, Viayna, Barrull, and Perulero, 2018). Biological sabotage in the form of anthrax and glanders was undertaken on behalf of the Imperial German government during World War I (1914–1918), with indifferent results (Jenkins, Baingana, Ahmad, McDaid, and

Atun, 2011; Johnson, Alvarez-Pasquin, Bijl, Franco, Gaillat, Clara, and Weinke, 2015). The Geneva Protocol of 1925 prohibited the use of chemical and biological weapons (Purevdawa, Moon, Baigalmaa, Davaajav, Smith, and Vermund, 1997; Ramesh, Malla, Raju, Sehgal, Ganguly, Mahajan, and Dilawari, 1990). With the onset of World War II, the Ministry of Supply in the United Kingdom established a bio weaponry program at Porton Down, headed by the microbiologist Paul Fildes (Jenkins, Baingana, Ahmad, McDaid, and Atun, 2011; Johnson, Alvarez-Pasquin, Bijl, Franco, Gaillat, Clara, and Weinke, 2015). The research was championed by Winston Churchill and soon tularemia, anthrax, brucellosis, and botulism toxins had been effectively weaponized (Krieger, 2001a, b; Lemma, 1969; Liu, Maniadakis, Gray, and Rayner, 2002; López, Torné, Franco, San-Martin, Viayna, Barrull, and Perulero, 2018). In particular, Gruinard Island in Scotland, was contaminated with anthrax during a series of extensive tests for the next 56 years (Narrod, Zinsstag, and Tiongco, 2012; Nascimento and de Oliveira, 2014; O'Brien, Lahue, Caro, and Davidson, 2007). Although the UK never offensively used the biological weapons it developed, its program was the first to successfully weaponize a variety of deadly pathogens and bring them into industrial production (Pal, Kerorsa, Marami, and Kandi, 2020; Paterson, Otte, Slingenbergh, Wint, and Rogers, 2000; Pearce and Merletti, 2006). Other nations, notably France and Japan, had begun their own biological weapons programs (Buckley, 1984; Budke, Jiamin, Qian, and Torgerson, 2005; Bundy, Arámbulo III, and Grey, 1983; Buzby and Roberts, 2009).

When the United States entered the war, allied resources were pooled at the request of the British, and the U.S. established a large research program and industrial complex at Fort Detrick, Maryland in 1942 under the direction of George W. Merck (Ozmen, Kurşun, and Ozcelik, 2005; Paarlberg, Hillberg, Lee, and Mathews, 2008; Paisley, Vraa-Andersen, Dybkjaer, Møller, Christensen, Mousing, and Agger, 1993). The biological and chemical weapons developed during that period were tested at the Dugway Proving Grounds in Utah (Hart and Halden, 2020; Häsler, Howe, and Stärk, 2011; Henschke, Kamper, and Maher, 2015; Hochberg, 1992). Soon there were facilities for the mass production of anthrax spores, brucellosis, and botulism toxins (Bausch and Schwarz, 2014; Bausch et al., 2001; Benner, Carabin, Sánchez-Serrano, Budke, and Carmena, 2010). This was despite the fact that the war was over before these weapons could be of much operational use (Saleha, 1991; Sibert, Rigaud, Delavierre, and Labat, 2010; Skrepnek and Skrepnek, 2004; Sloane, 2009; Sockett, 1993). The most notorious program of the period was run by the secret Imperial Japanese Army Unit 731 during the war, based at Pingfan in Manchuria and commanded by Lieutenant General Shirō Ishii (Fenichel, 2013; Fenichel et al., 2011; Fogel, 1994). This unit did research on bio weaponry, conducted often fatal human experiments on prisoners, and produced biological weapons for combat use (Abegunde and Stanciole, 2008; Abramowitz, Lacau Saint Guily, Moyal-Barracco, Bergeron, Borne, Dahlab, and Bénard, 2018).

Although the Japanese effort lacked the technological sophistication of the American or British programs, it far outstripped them in its widespread application and indiscriminate brutality (Perry and Randolph, 1999; Philipson, 2000; Philipson and Posner, 1996; Pongchaiyakul, Songpattanasilp, and Taechakraichana, 2008). Biological weapons were used against Chinese soldiers and civilians in several military campaigns (Yi-Xin and Manderson, 2005; Zadoks, 2008; Zhan, Li, Wang, Sun, Geng, Xiong, and de Hoog, 2015; Zhang, Song, Cai, and Zhou, 2008). In 1940, the Japanese Army Air Force bombed Ningbo with ceramic bombs full of fleas carrying the bubonic plague (Rogers, Carolin, Vaught, and Compton, 2011; Ronohardjo and Rastiko, 1982; Sachs, 2001; Sachs and Malaney, 2002). Many of these operations were ineffective due to inefficient delivery systems, although up to 400,000 people may have died (Arredondo and Zúñiga, 2006; Backer, van Roermund, Fischer, van Asseldonk, and Bergevoet, 2015; Bartsch, Hotez, Hertenstein, Diemert, Zapf, Bottazzi, and Lee, 2016). During the Zhejiang-Jiangxi Campaign in 1942, around 1,700 Japanese troops died out of a total 10,000 Japanese soldiers who fell ill with disease when their own biological weapons attack rebounded on their own forces (Chen, Li, Hsieh, Chang, Lee, Lee, and Ko, 2012; Conover, Pitt, Kessler, DuBow, and Sanborn, 1995; Crump, Murdoch, and Baker, 2001). During the final months of World War II, Japan planned to use plague as a biological weapon against U.S. civilians in San Diego, California, during Operation Cherry Blossoms at Night (Daily, and Ehrlich, 1996; Deogaonkar, Hutubessy, Van Der Putten, Evers, and Jit, 2012; Dorn, 1992; Ducrotoy, Bertu, Ocholi, Gusi, Bryssinckx, Welburn, and Moriyon, 2014). The plan was set to launch on 22 September 1945, but it was not executed because of Japan's surrender on 15 August 1945 (Weycker, Edelsberg, Oster, and Tino, 2005; Wu, Perrings, Kinzig, Collins, Minteer, and Daszak, 2017; Yach, Stuckler, and Brownell, 2006).

Biological weapons are difficult to detect, economical, and easy to use, making them appealing to terrorists (Howe, Häsler, and Stärk, 2013; Howe et al., 2012). The cost of a biological weapon is estimated to be about 0.05% the cost of a conventional weapon in order to produce similar numbers of mass casualties per kilometer square (Foxman, 2002; Garner, Whan, Gard, and Phillips, 2001; Gayle and Hill, 2001; Gottstein, Pozio, and Nöckler, 2009). Moreover, their production is very easy as common technology can be used to produce biological warfare, like that used in the production of vaccines, foods, spray devices, beverages, and antibiotics (Raut, 2004; Rehm, Mathers, Popova, Thavorncharoensap, Teerawattananon, and Patra, 2009; Rich and Perry, 2011). A major factor in biological warfare that attracts terrorists is that they can easily escape before the government agencies or secret agencies have even started their investigation (Uusküla, Müürsepp, Kawai, Raag, Jürisson, and Pillsbury, 2013; Vanni, Karnon, Madan, White, Edmunds, Foss, and Legood, 2011). This is because the potential organism has an incubation period of 3 to 7 days, after which the results begin to appear, thereby giving terrorists a lead (Moné, Ibikounlé, Massougbodji, and Mouahid, 2010; Morand, 2004; Moro, Budke, Schantz, Vasquez, Santivanez, and Villavicencio, 2011).

Entomological warfare is a type of biological warfare that uses insects to attack the enemy (Tapia, 2003; Torgerson and Dowling, 2001; Torgerson, Carmona, and Bonifacino, 2000; Uddin Khan, Atanasova, Krueger, Ramirez, and Gray, 2013). The concept has existed for centuries, and research and development have continued into the modern era (Bergevoet, Van Schaik, Veling, Backus, and Franken, 2009; Binder, 1988; Bolos, Bacarea, and Marusteri, 2011). Entomological warfare has been used in battle by Japan and several other nations have developed and been accused of using an entomological warfare program (Suhrcke, Stuckler, Suk, Desai, Senek, McKee, and Rechel, 2011; Šumilo, Bormane, Asokliene, Vasilenko, Golovljova, Avsic-Zupanc, and Randolph, 2008). This type of war may employ insects in a direct attack or as vectors to deliver a biological agent, such as plague (Markos and Abdela, 2016; Martin and Shepherd, 2009; McGuinness, McGlynn, Johnson, MacIntyre, Batty, Burns, and McGinty, 2012). Essentially, entomological warfare exists in three varieties (Espinoza, Terashima, Herrera-Velit, and Marcos, 2010; Ezzati, Vander Hoorn, Lawes, Leach, James, Lopez, and Murray, 2005). One type involves infecting insects with a pathogen and then dispersing the insects over target areas (Eaton and Groopman, 2013; Eckelman, Sherman, and MacNeill, 2018; Egger, 2011; Elbe, 2007; Ernst and Hay, 1994). The insects then act as a vector, infecting any person or animal they might bite. Another type is a direct insect attack against crops (Acemoglu and Johnson, 2007; Adda, 2016; Alloul, Sauriol, Kennedy, Laurier, Tessier, Novosel, and Contandriopoulos, 1998). The insect may not be infected with any pathogen but instead represents a threat to agriculture (Amuna and Zotor, 2008; Aral, Holmes, Padian, and Cates, 1996; Arbabi, Nezami, Hooshyar, and Delavari, 2018). The final method uses uninfected insects, such as bees, wasps, etc., to directly attack the enemy (Peckham, 2013; Perrings et al., 2002, 2014).

CHAPTER 2 SUMMARY

This chapter has considered some of the common origins of disease pandemics. Some of the factors that have been implicated include climate change, population growth, culture, lifestyle, and bio weaponry. Throughout, the chapter makes it clear that the threat is ever-present and that the risks are increasing with global travel and the interconnected nature of our contemporary existence. In the next chapter, we consider the progression of disease epidemics and how this impacts on their effects on the community.

Chapter 3

The Progress of a Disease Epidemic

CONTENTS

The stages through which a disease pandemic passes are important in defining it and the impact that it has on the community. Hence, the third chapter in this book will consider the various stages of progression of disease epidemics. This chapter must be read, bearing in mind the fact that the stages are not set in stone and may overlap or even be skipped over in some instances. Nevertheless, the broad categorizations that are summarized in this chapter help us better understand the nature of a disease epidemic. Specifically, the chapter will explore the inception or origin, spread, and virulence, introduction to novel locations, changes in host susceptibility, and finally, community immunity or what is now being referred to as "herd immunity." By the end of this chapter, the reader should have an idea of how disease epidemics arise and spread in the community.

3.1. INCEPTION AND ORIGIN OF A DISEASE EPIDEMIC

The World Health Organization (WHO) pandemic phases were developed in 1999 and revised in 2005 (Borghol, Suderman, McArdle, Racine, Hallett, Pembrey, and Szyf, 2012; Brandes, 2008; Brown, Lipscomb, and Snyder, 2001). The phases are applicable to the entire world and provide a global framework to aid countries in pandemic preparedness and response planning (Bwire, Munier, Ouedraogo, Heyerdahl, Komakech, Kagirita, and Makumbi, 2017; Canali, Aragrande, Angheben, Capelli, Drigo, Gobbi, and Cassini, 2020). In this revision, WHO has retained the use of a six-phased approach for easy incorporation of new recommendations and approaches into existing national preparedness and response plans (Armelagos, Brown, and Turner, 2005; Arokiasamy and Krishnan, 1994; Arora, 2001, 2005; Arredondo and Zúñiga, 2004). The grouping and description of pandemic phases have been revised to make them easier to understand, more precise, and based upon observable phenomena (Oleś, Gudowska-Nowak, and Kleczkowski, 2012; Otte, Nugent, and McLeod, 2004; Ozawa, Portnoy, Getaneh, Clark, Knoll, Bishai, and Patwardhan, 2016). Phases 1–3 correlate with preparedness, including capacity development and response planning activities, while Phases 4–6 clearly signal the need for response and mitigation efforts (Bonds, Keenan, Rohani, and Sachs, 2010; Boni, Galvani, Wickelgren, and Malani, 2013; Bonovas and Nikolopoulos, 2012). In Figure 3.1, we see the estimated timelines of the HIV/AIDS pandemic. However, many question whether such maps are accurate given the fact that many as-yet-unknown diseases exist in the community (Kim and Goldie, 2008;

Klein, Laxminarayan, Smith, and Gilligan, 2007; Klepac, Laxminarayan, and Grenfell, 2011).

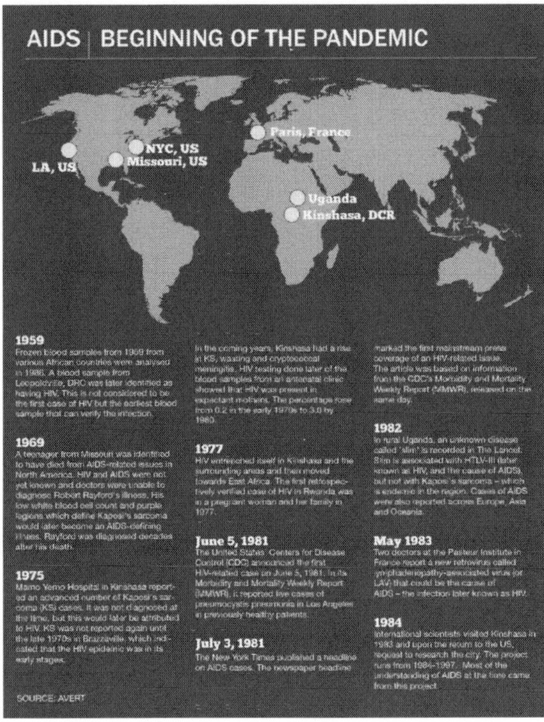

Figure 3.1. Estimated timeline of the HIV/AIDS pandemic.

Source: Avert via Aljazeera.

Furthermore, periods after the first pandemic wave are elaborated to facilitate post-pandemic recovery (St George, 1986; Steben and Duarte-Franco, 2007; Stehr-Green and Schantz, 1987; Stuckler, 2008; Stuckler and Siegel, 2011). Some of the notable changes include the use of phases as a planning tool (Poundstone, Strathdee, and Celentano, 2004; Pritchett, Thilmany, and Johnson, 2005; Pugliatti, Beghi, Forsgren, Ekman, and Sobocki, 2007). The new phases are simpler, more precise, and based on verifiable phenomena (Casamassimo, Thikkurissy, Edelstein, and Maiorini, 2009; Castro, Wilson, and Bloom, 2017). However, the phases only loosely correspond to pandemic risk and therefore local conditions must be carefully studied when planning and implementing a response to any pandemic (Yi-Xin and Manderson, 2005; Zadoks, 2008; Zhan, Li, Wang, Sun, Geng, Xiong, and de Hoog, 2015; Zhang, Song, Cai, and Zhou, 2008).

Authorities are required to identify sustained human-to-human transmission as a key event (Weycker, Edelsberg, Oster, and Tino, 2005; Wu, Perrings, Kinzig, Collins, Minteer, and Daszak, 2017; Yach, Stuckler, and Brownell, 2006). When using the guidelines, it is better to distinguish between time for preparedness and response (Uusküla, Müürsepp, Kawai, Raag, Jürisson, and Pillsbury, 2013; Vanni, Karnon, Madan, White, Edmunds, Foss, and Legood, 2011). This allows for a much more coherent and coordinated response to the disease pandemic (Tapia, 2003; Torgerson and Dowling, 2001; Torgerson, Carmona, and Bonifacino, 2000; Uddin Khan, Atanasova, Krueger, Ramirez, and Gray, 2013).

The WHO guidelines include the post-peak and post-pandemic periods for recovery activities in order to provide an overall strategic view of the phenomena (Suhrcke, Stuckler, Suk, Desai, Senek, McKee, and Rechel, 2011; Šumilo, Bormane, Asokliene, Vasilenko, Golovljova, Avsic-Zupanc, and Randolph, 2008). Nevertheless, it is important to note that the new phases are not designed to predict what will happen during a pandemic or even suggest that the pandemics are always going to proceed in numerical order (St George, 1986; Steben and Duarte-Franco, 2007; Stehr-Green and Schantz, 1987; Stuckler, 2008; Stuckler and Siegel, 2011). Each locality will have its own trajectory of the pandemic which may differ from others or even the set format (Saleha, 1991; Sibert, Rigaud, Delavierre, and Labat, 2010; Skrepnek and Skrepnek, 2004; Sloane, 2009; Sockett, 1993). Instead, the guidelines merely provide an overview of how pandemics have traditionally emerged and progressed (Rogers, Carolin, Vaught, and Compton, 2011; Ronohardjo and Rastiko, 1982; Sachs, 2001; Sachs and Malaney, 2002).

In nature, influenza viruses circulate continuously among animals, especially birds (Raut, 2004; Rehm, Mathers, Popova, Thavorncharoensap, Teerawattananon, and Patra, 2009; Rich and Perry, 2011). Even though such viruses might theoretically develop into pandemic viruses, in Phase 1 no viruses circulating among animals have been reported to cause infections in humans (Purevdawa, Moon, Baigalmaa, Davaajav, Smith, and Vermund, 1997; Ramesh, Malla, Raju, Sehgal, Ganguly, Mahajan, and Dilawari, 1990). Background Surveillance of infectious diseases is done in many countries (Poundstone, Strathdee, and Celentano, 2004; Pritchett, Thilmany, and Johnson, 2005; Pugliatti, Beghi, Forsgren, Ekman, and Sobocki, 2007). The aims of such surveillance include the detection of epidemics (Perry and Randolph, 1999; Philipson, 2000; Philipson and Posner, 1996; Pongchaiyakul, Songpattanasilp, and Taechakraichana, 2008). For example, the possibility of detecting an epidemic in its early stage using a simple method is evaluated for several infectious diseases (Peckham, 2013; Perrings et al., 2002, 2014). The aim of such surveillance includes detection of epidemics, especially detection in the early stage, essential for the control of epidemics of infectious diseases (Pal, Kerorsa, Marami, and Kandi, 2020; Paterson, Otte, Slingenbergh, Wint, and Rogers, 2000; Pearce and Merletti, 2006). Epidemics generally begin in small areas and subsequently spread widely (Ozmen, Kurşun, and Ozcelik, 2005; Paarlberg, Hillberg, Lee, and Mathews, 2008; Paisley, Vraa-Andersen, Dybkjaer, Møller, Christensen, Mousing, and Agger, 1993). In order to detect an epidemic in its early stage, observation of the data for small areas is important (Oleś, Gudowska-Nowak, and Kleczkowski, 2012; Otte, Nugent, and McLeod, 2004; Ozawa, Portnoy, Getaneh, Clark, Knoll, Bishai, and Patwardhan, 2016).

Many epidemiological and statistical studies have investigated the detection of epidemics through surveillance (Narrod, Zinsstag, and Tiongco, 2012; Nascimento and de Oliveira, 2014; O'Brien, Lahue, Caro, and Davidson, 2007). These investigations have mainly focused on epidemics of influenza-like illnesses in a large area (whole country), while epidemics in small areas (such as city, town) and of other infectious diseases have received insufficient attention (Moné, Ibikounlé, Massougbodji, and Mouahid, 2010; Morand, 2004; Moro, Budke, Schantz, Vasquez, Santivanez, and Villavicencio, 2011). Several methods for detecting and forecasting epidemics, such as time series analysis, are often applied (Markos and Abdela, 2016; Martin and Shepherd, 2009; McGuinness, McGlynn, Johnson, MacIntyre, Batty, Burns, and McGinty, 2012). Some methods require strict assumptions in their underlying models and are too complicated to be applied to the data for small areas (Krieger, 2001a, b; Lemma, 1969; Liu, Maniadakis, Gray, and Rayner, 2002; López, Torné, Franco, San-Martin, Viayna, Barrull, and Perulero, 2018). Many researchers are of the view that simple methods for detecting epidemics would be more practical for public health activities (Kim and Goldie, 2008; Klein, Laxminarayan, Smith, and Gilligan, 2007; Klepac, Laxminarayan, and Grenfell, 2011).

Epidemic periods in health center areas are often determined according to their indices (Jenkins, Baingana, Ahmad, McDaid, and Atun, 2011; Johnson, Alvarez-Pasquin, Bijl, Franco, Gaillat, Clara, and Weinke, 2015). Researchers tend to assume that an epidemic began in the week when its index exceeded a certain value (Howe, Häsler, and Stärk, 2013; Howe et al., 2012). This is the critical value for the onset of an epidemic (Hart and Halden, 2020; Häsler, Howe, and Stärk, 2011; Henschke, Kamper, and Maher, 2015; Hochberg, 1992). Another assumption is that the epidemic ended the week before indices in four successive weeks were lower than another given value (Foxman, 2002; Garner, Whan, Gard, and Phillips, 2001; Gayle and Hill, 2001; Gottstein, Pozio, and Nöckler, 2009). This is the critical value for the end of an epidemic (Fenichel, 2013; Fenichel et al., 2011; Fogel, 1994). There are many triggers that must be put in place at this early stage in order to avoid the spread and increased virulence that we will explore in the next section.

3.2. SPREAD AND INCREASE VIRULENCE OF A DISEASE EPIDEMIC

The second phase of a disease epidemic is characterized by the animal virus circulating among domesticated or wild animals (Espinoza, Terashima, Herrera-Velit, and Marcos, 2010; Ezzati, Vander Hoorn, Lawes, Leach, James, Lopez, and Murray, 2005). At this stage, the pandemic is known to have caused infection in humans, and is therefore considered a potential pandemic threat (Eaton and Groopman, 2013; Eckelman, Sherman, and MacNeill, 2018; Egger, 2011; Elbe, 2007; Ernst and Hay, 1994). Virulence is a pathogen's or microbe's ability to infect or damage a host (Chen, Li, Hsieh, Chang, Lee, Lee, and Ko, 2012; Conover, Pitt, Kessler, DuBow, and Sanborn, 1995; Crump, Murdoch, and Baker, 2001).

In the context of gene for gene systems, say for example as in plants; virulence refers to a pathogen's ability to infect a resistant host (Casamassimo, Thikkurissy, Edelstein, and Maiorini, 2009; Castro, Wilson, and Bloom, 2017). In most other contexts, especially in animal systems, virulence refers to the degree of damage caused by a microbe to its host (Bwire, Munier, Ouedraogo, Heyerdahl, Komakech, Kagirita, and Makumbi, 2017; Canali, Aragrande, Angheben, Capelli, Drigo, Gobbi, and Cassini, 2020). The pathogenicity of an organism or its ability to cause disease is determined by its virulence factors (Buckley, 1984; Budke, Jiamin, Qian, and Torgerson, 2005; Bundy, Arámbulo III, and Grey, 1983; Buzby and Roberts, 2009). Virulent can describe either disease severity or a pathogen's infectivity (Borghol, Suderman, McArdle, Racine, Hallett, Pembrey, and Szyf, 2012; Brandes, 2008; Brown, Lipscomb, and Snyder, 2001). Figure 3.2 highlights the trajectories of the Spanish Flue as a case in point.

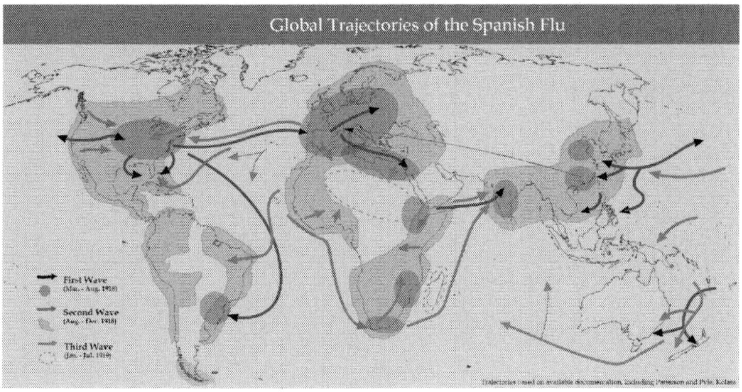

Figure 3.2. Global trajectories of the Spanish flue.

Source: Africa Center for Strategic Studies.

In ecology, virulence is the host's parasite-induced loss of fitness (Bonds, Keenan, Rohani, and Sachs, 2010; Boni, Galvani, Wickelgren, and Malani, 2013; Bonovas and Nikolopoulos, 2012). Virulence can be understood in terms of proximate causes (Bergevoet, Van Schaik, Veling, Backus, and Franken, 2009; Binder, 1988; Bolos, Bacarea, and Marusteri, 2011). This refers to those specific traits of the pathogen that help make the host ill and ultimate causes the evolutionary pressures that lead to virulent traits occurring in a pathogen strain (Bausch and Schwarz, 2014; Bausch et al., 2001; Benner, Carabin, Sánchez-Serrano, Budke, and Carmena, 2010). The ability of bacteria to cause disease is described in terms of the number of infecting bacteria, the route of entry into the body, the effects of host defense mechanisms, and intrinsic characteristics of the bacteria called virulence factors (Arredondo and Zúñiga, 2006; Backer, van Roermund, Fischer, van Asseldonk, and Bergevoet, 2015; Bartsch, Hotez, Hertenstein, Diemert, Zapf, Bottazzi, and Lee, 2016). Many virulence factors are so-called effector proteins that are injected into the host cells by special secretion machines such as the type 3 secretion system (Armelagos, Brown, and Turner, 2005; Arokiasamy and Krishnan, 1994; Arora, 2001, 2005; Arredondo and Zúñiga, 2004). Host-mediated pathogenesis are often important because the host can respond aggressively to infection with the result that host defense mechanisms do damage to host tissues while the infection is being countered (Amuna and Zotor, 2008; Aral, Holmes, Padian, and Cates, 1996; Arbabi, Nezami, Hooshyar, and Delavari, 2018).

The virulence factors of bacteria are typically proteins or other molecules that are synthesized by enzymes (Acemoglu and Johnson, 2007;

Adda, 2016; Alloul, Sauriol, Kennedy, Laurier, Tessier, Novosel, and Contandriopoulos, 1998). These proteins are coded by genes in chromosomal DNA, bacteriophage DNA or plasmids (Abegunde and Stanciole, 2008; Abramowitz, Lacau Saint Guily, Moyal-Barracco, Bergeron, Borne, Dahlab, and Bénard, 2018). Certain bacteria employ mobile genetic elements and horizontal gene transfer (Ozmen, Kurşun, and Ozcelik, 2005; Paarlberg, Hillberg, Lee, and Mathews, 2008; Paisley, Vraa-Andersen, Dybkjaer, Møller, Christensen, Mousing, and Agger, 1993). Therefore, strategies to combat certain bacterial infections by targeting these specific virulence factors and mobile genetic elements have been proposed (Bonds, Keenan, Rohani, and Sachs, 2010; Boni, Galvani, Wickelgren, and Malani, 2013; Bonovas and Nikolopoulos, 2012). Bacteria use quorum sensing to synchronize the release of the molecules. These are all proximate causes of morbidity in the host (Espinoza, Terashima, Herrera-Velit, and Marcos, 2010; Ezzati, Vander Hoorn, Lawes, Leach, James, Lopez, and Murray, 2005). There are a several methods through which bacteria can cause infection (Buckley, 1984; Budke, Jiamin, Qian, and Torgerson, 2005; Bundy, Arámbulo III, and Grey, 1983; Buzby and Roberts, 2009).

The first method is what is known as adhesion (Bwire, Munier, Ouedraogo, Heyerdahl, Komakech, Kagirita, and Makumbi, 2017; Canali, Aragrande, Angheben, Capelli, Drigo, Gobbi, and Cassini, 2020). Many bacteria must first bind to host cell surfaces (Yi-Xin and Manderson, 2005; Zadoks, 2008; Zhan, Li, Wang, Sun, Geng, Xiong, and de Hoog, 2015; Zhang, Song, Cai, and Zhou, 2008). Many bacterial and host molecules that are involved in the adhesion of bacteria to host cells have been identified (Pal, Kerorsa, Marami, and Kandi, 2020; Paterson, Otte, Slingenbergh, Wint, and Rogers, 2000; Pearce and Merletti, 2006). Often, the host cell receptors for bacteria are essential proteins for other functions (Jenkins, Baingana, Ahmad, McDaid, and Atun, 2011; Johnson, Alvarez-Pasquin, Bijl, Franco, Gaillat, Clara, and Weinke, 2015). Due to the presence of mucous lining and of anti-microbial substances around some host cells, it is difficult for certain pathogens to establish direct contact-adhesion (Abegunde and Stanciole, 2008; Abramowitz, Lacau Saint Guily, Moyal-Barracco, Bergeron, Borne, Dahlab, and Bénard, 2018). The second method is known as colonization (Kim and Goldie, 2008; Klein, Laxminarayan, Smith, and Gilligan, 2007; Klepac, Laxminarayan, and Grenfell, 2011). Some virulent bacteria produce special proteins that allow them to colonize parts of the host body (Chen, Li, Hsieh, Chang, Lee, Lee, and Ko, 2012; Conover, Pitt, Kessler, DuBow, and Sanborn, 1995; Crump, Murdoch, and Baker, 2001). Helicobacter pylori is able to survive in the acidic environment of the human stomach by producing the enzyme urease (Weycker, Edelsberg, Oster, and Tino, 2005; Wu, Perrings, Kinzig, Collins, Minteer, and Daszak, 2017; Yach, Stuckler, and Brownell, 2006). Colonization of the stomach lining by this bacterium can lead to gastric ulcers and cancer (Perry and Randolph, 1999; Philipson, 2000; Philipson and Posner, 1996; Pongchaiyakul, Songpattanasilp, and Taechakraichana, 2008). The virulence of various strains of Helicobacter pylori tends to correlate with the level of production of urease (Uusküla, Müürsepp, Kawai, Raag, Jürisson, and Pillsbury, 2013; Vanni, Karnon, Madan, White, Edmunds, Foss, and Legood, 2011).

The third modality is that of invasion (St George, 1986; Steben and Duarte-Franco, 2007; Stehr-Green and Schantz, 1987; Stuckler, 2008; Stuckler and Siegel, 2011). Some virulent bacteria produce proteins that either disrupt host cell membranes or stimulate their own endocytosis or macro-pinocytosis into host cells (Acemoglu and Johnson, 2007; Adda, 2016; Alloul, Sauriol, Kennedy, Laurier, Tessier, Novosel, and Contandriopoulos, 1998). These virulence factors allow the bacteria to enter host cells and facilitate entry into the body across epithelial tissue layers at the body surface (Amuna and Zotor, 2008; Aral, Holmes, Padian, and Cates, 1996; Arbabi, Nezami, Hooshyar, and Delavari, 2018). The 4th approach is through immune response inhibitors. Many bacteria produce virulence factors that inhibit the host's immune system defenses (Krieger, 2001a, b; Lemma, 1969; Liu, Maniadakis, Gray, and Rayner, 2002; López, Torné, Franco, San-Martin, Viayna, Barrull, and Perulero, 2018). For example, a common bacterial strategy is to produce proteins that bind host antibodies (Armelagos, Brown, and Turner, 2005; Arokiasamy and Krishnan, 1994; Arora, 2001, 2005; Arredondo and Zúñiga, 2004). The polysaccharide capsule of Streptococcus pneumoniae inhibits phagocytosis of the bacterium by host immune cells (Poundstone, Strathdee, and Celentano, 2004; Pritchett, Thilmany, and Johnson, 2005; Pugliatti, Beghi, Forsgren, Ekman, and Sobocki, 2007). The 5th modality is via toxins (Suhrcke, Stuckler, Suk, Desai, Senek, McKee, and Rechel, 2011; Šumilo, Bormane, Asokliene, Vasilenko, Golovljova, Avsic-Zupanc, and Randolph, 2008). Many virulence factors are proteins made by bacteria that poison host cells and cause tissue damage (Bergevoet, Van Schaik, Veling, Backus, and Franken, 2009; Binder, 1988; Bolos, Bacarea, and Marusteri, 2011). For example, there are many food poisoning toxins produced by bacteria that can contaminate human foods (Arredondo and Zúñiga, 2006; Backer, van Roermund, Fischer, van Asseldonk, and Bergevoet, 2015; Bartsch, Hotez, Hertenstein, Diemert, Zapf, Bottazzi, and

Lee, 2016). Some of these can remain in "spoiled" food even after cooking and cause illness when the contaminated food is consumed (Howe, Häsler, and Stärk, 2013; Howe et al., 2012). Other bacterial toxins are chemically altered and inactivated by the heat of cooking (Raut, 2004; Rehm, Mathers, Popova, Thavorncharoensap, Teerawattananon, and Patra, 2009; Rich and Perry, 2011).

Virus virulence factors allow it to replicate, modify host defenses, and spread within the host, and they are toxic to the host (Hart and Halden, 2020; Häsler, Howe, and Stärk, 2011; Henschke, Kamper, and Maher, 2015; Hochberg, 1992). They determine whether infection occurs and how severe the resulting viral disease symptoms are (Markos and Abdela, 2016; Martin and Shepherd, 2009; McGuinness, McGlynn, Johnson, MacIntyre, Batty, Burns, and McGinty, 2012). Viruses often require receptor proteins on host cells to which they specifically bind (Foxman, 2002; Garner, Whan, Gard, and Phillips, 2001; Gayle and Hill, 2001; Gottstein, Pozio, and Nöckler, 2009). Typically, these host cell proteins are endocytosed and the bound virus then enters the host cell (Eaton and Groopman, 2013; Eckelman, Sherman, and MacNeill, 2018; Egger, 2011; Elbe, 2007; Ernst and Hay, 1994). Virulent viruses such as HIV, which causes AIDS, have mechanisms for evading host defenses (Moné, Ibikounlé, Massougbodji, and Mouahid, 2010; Morand, 2004; Moro, Budke, Schantz, Vasquez, Santivanez, and Villavicencio, 2011). HIV infects T-Helper Cells, which leads to a reduction of the adaptive immune response of the host and eventually leads to an immunocompromised state (Oleś, Gudowska-Nowak, and Kleczkowski, 2012; Otte, Nugent, and McLeod, 2004; Ozawa, Portnoy, Getaneh, Clark, Knoll, Bishai, and Patwardhan, 2016). Death results from opportunistic infections secondary to disruption of the immune system caused by AIDS (Rogers, Carolin, Vaught, and Compton, 2011; Ronohardjo and Rastiko, 1982; Sachs, 2001; Sachs and Malaney, 2002).

Some viral virulence factors confer the ability to replicate during the defensive inflammation responses of the host, such as during virus-induced fever (Bausch and Schwarz, 2014; Bausch et al., 2001; Benner, Carabin, Sánchez-Serrano, Budke, and Carmena, 2010). Many viruses can exist inside a host for long periods during which little damage is done (Purevdawa, Moon, Baigalmaa, Davaajav, Smith, and Vermund, 1997; Ramesh, Malla, Raju, Sehgal, Ganguly, Mahajan, and Dilawari, 1990). Extremely virulent strains can eventually evolve by mutation and natural selection within the virus population inside a host (Borghol, Suderman, McArdle, Racine, Hallett, Pembrey, and Szyf, 2012; Brandes, 2008; Brown, Lipscomb, and

Snyder, 2001). The term "neurovirulent" is used for viruses such as rabies and herpes simplex which can invade the nervous system and cause disease there (Tapia, 2003; Torgerson and Dowling, 2001; Torgerson, Carmona, and Bonifacino, 2000; Uddin Khan, Atanasova, Krueger, Ramirez, and Gray, 2013). Extensively studied model organisms of virulent viruses include virus T4 and other T-even bacteriophages which infect Escherichia coli and a number of related bacteria (Saleha, 1991; Sibert, Rigaud, Delavierre, and Labat, 2010; Skrepnek and Skrepnek, 2004; Sloane, 2009; Sockett, 1993).

According to evolutionary medicine, optimal virulence increases with horizontal transmission (between non-relatives) and decreases with vertical transmission (from parent to child) (Peckham, 2013; Perrings et al., 2002, 2014). This is because the fitness of the host is bound to the fitness in vertical transmission but is not so bound in horizontal transmission (Daily, and Ehrlich, 1996; Deogaonkar, Hutubessy, Van Der Putten, Evers, and Jit, 2012; Dorn, 1992; Ducrotoy, Bertu, Ocholi, Gusi, Bryssinckx, Welburn, and Moriyon, 2014). Theory predicts that selection for pathogen virulence and horizontal transmission is highest at the onset of an epidemic but decreases thereafter, as the epidemic depletes the pool of susceptible hosts (Fenichel, 2013; Fenichel et al., 2011; Fogel, 1994). Understanding and predicting the conditions under which pathogens evolve towards higher levels of virulence (pathogen-induced host mortality) is a major challenge in the control of infectious diseases (Narrod, Zinsstag, and Tiongco, 2012; Nascimento and de Oliveira, 2014; O'Brien, Lahue, Caro, and Davidson, 2007). Nevertheless, the theoretical understanding of virulence evolution is often based on several major simplifying assumptions (Casamassimo, Thikkurissy, Edelstein, and Maiorini, 2009; Castro, Wilson, and Bloom, 2017). In particular, the classical adaptive dynamics framework assumes that mutations are rare and thus that evolution occurs on a much slower time scale than epidemiological dynamics (Abegunde and Stanciole, 2008; Abramowitz, Lacau Saint Guily, Moyal-Barracco, Bergeron, Borne, Dahlab, and Bénard, 2018).

In other words, adaptive dynamics theory relies on the assumption that there is very little amount of genetic variation in the pathogen population and that a single pathogen strain reaches an equilibrium before a new strain arises by mutation (Acemoglu and Johnson, 2007; Adda, 2016; Alloul, Sauriol, Kennedy, Laurier, Tessier, Novosel, and Contandriopoulos, 1998). However, ecological and evolutionary time scales may overlap when the amount of genetic variation is high (Amuna and Zotor, 2008; Aral, Holmes, Padian, and Cates, 1996; Arbabi, Nezami, Hooshyar, and Delavari, 2018). This is the case for many pathogens, and in particular for viruses with large mutation rates (Armelagos, Brown, and Turner, 2005; Arokiasamy and Krishnan, 1994; Arora, 2001, 2005; Arredondo and Zúñiga, 2004). The recurrent introduction of new mutants violates a major assumption of adaptive dynamics since many different strains may compete with each other before the system reaches a new endemic equilibrium (Arredondo and Zúñiga, 2006; Backer, van Roermund, Fischer, van Asseldonk, and Bergevoet, 2015; Bartsch, Hotez, Hertenstein, Diemert, Zapf, Bottazzi, and Lee, 2016). Previous theoretical analyzes suggest that the outcome of this competition changes strikingly throughout an epidemic (Bausch and Schwarz, 2014; Bausch et al., 2001; Benner, Carabin, Sánchez-Serrano, Budke, and Carmena, 2010). This holds true even though selection can act against virulent mutants at the endemic equilibrium, there is a transitory phase during the early stage of the epidemic where the abundance of susceptible hosts can favor the more transmissible and aggressive strains (Bergevoet, Van Schaik, Veling, Backus, and Franken, 2009; Binder, 1988; Bolos, Bacarea, and Marusteri, 2011). The next section examines how disease epidemics are introduced to novel locations.

3.3. INTRODUCTION OF DISEASE EPIDEMICS TO NOVEL LOCATIONS

In Phase 3, an animal or human-animal virus has caused sporadic cases or small clusters of disease in people (Bonds, Keenan, Rohani, and Sachs, 2010; Boni, Galvani, Wickelgren, and Malani, 2013; Bonovas and Nikolopoulos, 2012). However, for the most part, this will not have resulted in human-to-human transmission, which is sufficiently high to sustain community-level outbreaks (Borghol, Suderman, McArdle, Racine, Hallett, Pembrey, and Szyf, 2012; Brandes, 2008; Brown, Lipscomb, and Snyder, 2001). Limited human-to-human transmission may occur under some circumstances (Buckley, 1984; Budke, Jiamin, Qian, and Torgerson, 2005; Bundy, Arámbulo III, and Grey, 1983; Buzby and Roberts, 2009). For example, infection may occur when there is close contact between an infected person and an unprotected caregiver (Bwire, Munier, Ouedraogo, Heyerdahl, Komakech, Kagirita, and Makumbi, 2017; Canali, Aragrande, Angheben, Capelli, Drigo, Gobbi, and Cassini, 2020). Nevertheless, limited transmission under such restricted circumstances does not indicate that the virus has gained the level of transmissibility among humans necessary to warrant a pandemic (Casamassimo, Thikkurissy, Edelstein, and Maiorini, 2009; Castro, Wilson, and Bloom, 2017). As the pandemic spreads, it starts to impact on the life span (see Figure 3.3 for examples in sub-Saharan Africa, which were impacted by the HIV/AIDS pandemic).

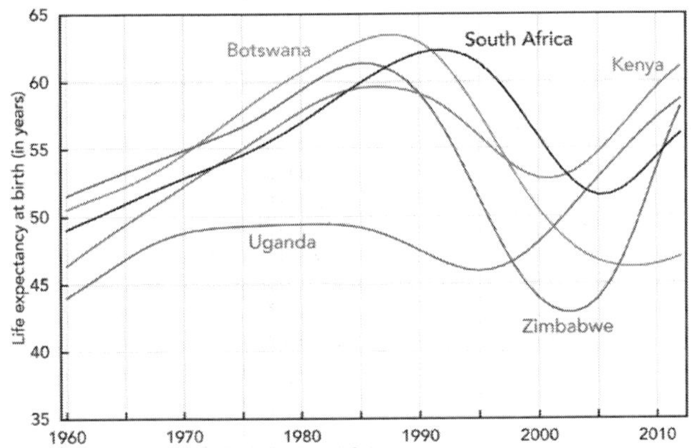

Figure 3.3. Impact of HIV/AIDS on mean life span among selected sub-Saharan countries.

Source: Wikipedia.

Human-to-human transmission or HHT is a particularly problematic epidemiologic vector, especially in case the disease is borne by individuals known as super-spreaders (Chen, Li, Hsieh, Chang, Lee, Lee, and Ko, 2012; Conover, Pitt, Kessler, DuBow, and Sanborn, 1995; Crump, Murdoch, and Baker, 2001). In these cases, the basic reproduction number of the virus, which is the average number of additional people that a single case will infect without any preventative measures, can be as high as 4 (Daily, and Ehrlich, 1996; Deogaonkar, Hutubessy, Van Der Putten, Evers, and Jit, 2012; Dorn, 1992; Ducrotoy, Bertu, Ocholi, Gusi, Bryssinckx, Welburn, and Moriyon, 2014). Indeed, inter-human transmission is a synonym for human-to-human transmission (Eaton and Groopman, 2013; Eckelman, Sherman, and MacNeill, 2018; Egger, 2011; Elbe, 2007; Ernst and Hay, 1994). The WHO designation of a pandemic hinges on the demonstrable fact that there is sustained human-to-human transmission in two regions of the world (Espinoza, Terashima, Herrera-Velit, and Marcos, 2010; Ezzati, Vander Hoorn, Lawes, Leach, James, Lopez, and Murray, 2005). When we speak of super-spreaders, it is important to mitigate against the possible social isolation that can face people who are considered to be "Patient Zero" or even "super spreaders" (Fenichel, 2013; Fenichel et al., 2011; Fogel, 1994). Often these are portrayed as being wicked threats to public health that may even face lynching in some parts of the world (Foxman, 2002; Garner, Whan, Gard, and Phillips, 2001; Gayle and Hill, 2001; Gottstein, Pozio, and Nöckler, 2009).

The transition into human-to-human transmission is a critical phase of the pandemic and many health professionals would prefer that this stage is prevented or curtailed as much as possible (Hart and Halden, 2020; Häsler, Howe, and Stärk, 2011; Henschke, Kamper, and Maher, 2015; Hochberg, 1992). Relevant pathogens may be viruses, bacteria, or fungi, and they may be spread through breathing, talking, coughing, sneezing, spraying of liquids, toilet flushing or any activities which generate aerosol particles or droplets or generate fomites, such as raising of dust (Howe, Häsler, and Stärk, 2013; Howe et al., 2012). A 2007 study showed that influenza virus was still active on stainless steel 24 hours after contamination. Though on hands it survives only for five minutes, the constant contact with steel almost certainly transmits infection. Transfer efficiency depends not only on the surface, but also on pathogen type (Jenkins, Baingana, Ahmad, McDaid, and Atun, 2011; Johnson, Alvarez-Pasquin, Bijl, Franco, Gaillat, Clara, and Weinke, 2015). For example, avian influenza survives on both porous and non-porous materials for 144 hours (Kim and Goldie, 2008; Klein, Laxminarayan, Smith, and Gilligan, 2007; Klepac, Laxminarayan, and Grenfell, 2011).

The pathogens may also be transmitted by poor use of cutlery or improper sanitation of dishes or bedlinen (Krieger, 2001a, b; Lemma, 1969; Liu, Maniadakis, Gray, and Rayner, 2002; López, Torné, Franco, San-Martin, Viayna, Barrull, and Perulero, 2018). Particularly problematic are toilet practices, which lead to the fecal-oral route (Markos and Abdela, 2016; Martin and Shepherd, 2009; McGuinness, McGlynn, Johnson, MacIntyre, Batty, Burns, and McGinty, 2012). Sexually Transmitted Diseases or STDs are by definition spread through this vector (Moné, Ibikounlé, Massougbodji, and Mouahid, 2010; Morand, 2004; Moro, Budke, Schantz, Vasquez, Santivanez, and Villavicencio, 2011). Infectious diseases, also known as infectiology, is a medical specialty dealing with the diagnosis and treatment of complex infections (Narrod, Zinsstag, and Tiongco, 2012; Nascimento and de Oliveira, 2014; O'Brien, Lahue, Caro, and Davidson, 2007). An infectious disease specialist's practice consists of managing nosocomial (healthcare-acquired) infections or community-acquired infections and is historically associated with travel medicine and tropical medicine (Oleś, Gudowska-Nowak, and Kleczkowski, 2012; Otte, Nugent, and McLeod, 2004; Ozawa, Portnoy, Getaneh, Clark, Knoll, Bishai, and Patwardhan,

2016). Infectious diseases specialists typically serve as consultants to other physicians in cases of complex infections, and often manage patients with HIV/AIDS and other forms of Immunodeficiency (Ozmen, Kurşun, and Ozcelik, 2005; Paarlberg, Hillberg, Lee, and Mathews, 2008; Paisley, Vraa-Andersen, Dybkjaer, Møller, Christensen, Mousing, and Agger, 1993).

Although many common infections are treated by physicians without formal expertise in infectious diseases, specialists may be consulted for cases where an infection is difficult to diagnose or manage (Pal, Kerorsa, Marami, and Kandi, 2020; Paterson, Otte, Slingenbergh, Wint, and Rogers, 2000; Pearce and Merletti, 2006). They may also be asked to help determine the cause of a fever of unknown origin. Specialists in infectious diseases can practice both in hospitals (inpatient) and clinics (outpatient) (Peckham, 2013; Perrings et al., 2002, 2014). In hospitals, specialists in infectious diseases help ensure the timely diagnosis and treatment of acute infections by recommending the appropriate diagnostic tests to identify the source of the infection and by recommending appropriate management such as prescribing antibiotics to treat bacterial infections (Perry and Randolph, 1999; Philipson, 2000; Philipson and Posner, 1996; Pongchaiyakul, Songpattanasilp, and Taechakraichana, 2008). For certain types of infections, the involvement of specialists in infectious diseases may improve patient outcomes (Poundstone, Strathdee, and Celentano, 2004; Pritchett, Thilmany, and Johnson, 2005; Pugliatti, Beghi, Forsgren, Ekman, and Sobocki, 2007). In clinics, specialists in infectious diseases can provide long-term care to patients with chronic infections such as HIV/AIDS (Purevdawa, Moon, Baigalmaa, Davaajav, Smith, and Vermund, 1997; Ramesh, Malla, Raju, Sehgal, Ganguly, Mahajan, and Dilawari, 1990).

Infectious diseases are historically associated with travel medicine and tropical medicine, as many diseases acquired in tropical and subtropical areas are infectious in nature (Raut, 2004; Rehm, Mathers, Popova, Thavorncharoensap, Teerawattananon, and Patra, 2009; Rich and Perry, 2011). Infectious diseases specialists employ a variety of diagnostic tests to help identify the pathogen that is causing an infection (Rogers, Carolin, Vaught, and Compton, 2011; Ronohardjo and Rastiko, 1982; Sachs, 2001; Sachs and Malaney, 2002). Common tests include Gram staining, blood cultures, serological tests, genotyping, and polymerase chain reaction (Saleha, 1991; Sibert, Rigaud, Delavierre, and Labat, 2010; Skrepnek and Skrepnek, 2004; Sloane, 2009; Sockett, 1993). Infectious diseases specialists employ a variety of antimicrobial agents to help treat infections (St George, 1986; Steben and Duarte-Franco, 2007; Stehr-Green and Schantz, 1987;

Stuckler, 2008; Stuckler and Siegel, 2011). The type of antimicrobial depends on the organism that is causing the infection (Suhrcke, Stuckler, Suk, Desai, Senek, McKee, and Rechel, 2011; Šumilo, Bormane, Asokliene, Vasilenko, Golovljova, Avsic-Zupanc, and Randolph, 2008). Antibiotics are used to treat bacterial infections; antiviral agents treat viral infections; and antifungal agents treat fungal infections (Tapia, 2003; Torgerson and Dowling, 2001; Torgerson, Carmona, and Bonifacino, 2000; Uddin Khan, Atanasova, Krueger, Ramirez, and Gray, 2013). The next section highlights how changes in the host susceptibility progresses in the pandemic.

3.4. CHANGES IN HOST SUSCEPTIBILITY TO DISEASE EPIDEMIC

Phase 4 of a disease epidemic is characterized by verified human-to-human transmission of the virus (or similar agent such as bacteria or protozoa) that is able to cause "community-level outbreaks (Uusküla, Müürsepp, Kawai, Raag, Jürisson, and Pillsbury, 2013; Vanni, Karnon, Madan, White, Edmunds, Foss, and Legood, 2011). The ability to cause sustained disease outbreaks in a community marks a significant upwards shift in the risk for a pandemic (Weycker, Edelsberg, Oster, and Tino, 2005; Wu, Perrings, Kinzig, Collins, Minteer, and Daszak, 2017; Yach, Stuckler, and Brownell, 2006). Any country that suspects or has verified such an event should urgently consult with WHO so that the situation can be jointly brought in for assessment and a decision made by the affected country if implementation of a rapid pandemic containment operation is warranted (Yi-Xin and Manderson, 2005; Zadoks, 2008; Zhan, Li, Wang, Sun, Geng, Xiong, and de Hoog, 2015; Zhang, Song, Cai, and Zhou, 2008). Phase 4 indicates a significant increase in risk of a pandemic but does not necessarily mean that a pandemic is a forgone conclusion (Casamassimo, Thikkurissy, Edelstein, and Maiorini, 2009; Castro, Wilson, and Bloom, 2017). Case fatalities are an important consideration for planners and healthcare professionals during this phase. In Figure 3.4, we see an overview of case fatalities in the COVID-19 outbreak, the most vulnerable being those who are older than 70 years.

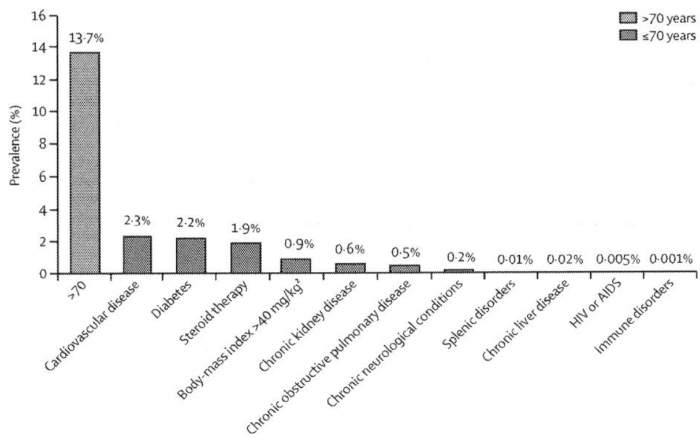

Figure 3.4. Estimating the excess 1-year mortality associated with COVID-19.

Source: The Lancet.

The susceptibility of populations or individuals is an important consideration, often referred to as the "host factor" (Fenichel, 2013; Fenichel et al., 2011; Fogel, 1994). Host factor is a medical term referring to the traits of an individual person or animal that affect susceptibility to disease, especially in comparison to other individuals (Daily, and Ehrlich, 1996; Deogaonkar, Hutubessy, Van Der Putten, Evers, and Jit, 2012; Dorn, 1992; Ducrotoy, Bertu, Ocholi, Gusi, Bryssinckx, Welburn, and Moriyon, 2014). The term arose in the context of infectious disease research, in contrast to "organism factors," such as the virulence and infectivity of a microbe (Peckham, 2013; Perrings et al., 2002, 2014). Host factors that may vary in a population and affect disease susceptibility can be innate or acquired. Some examples are: general health, psychological characteristics and attitude, nutritional state, social ties, previous exposure to the organism or related antigens, haplotype or other specific genetic differences of immune function, substance abuse, and race or ethnicity (Saleha, 1991; Sibert, Rigaud, Delavierre, and Labat, 2010; Skrepnek and Skrepnek, 2004; Sloane, 2009; Sockett, 1993).

The term "host factor" is now used in oncology and many other medical contexts related to individual differences of disease vulnerability (Tapia, 2003; Torgerson and Dowling, 2001; Torgerson, Carmona, and Bonifacino, 2000; Uddin Khan, Atanasova, Krueger, Ramirez, and Gray, 2013). Susceptible individuals or "susceptible" have been exposed to neither the wild strain of the disease nor a vaccination against it, and thus have not developed immunity (Borghol, Suderman, McArdle, Racine, Hallett, Pembrey, and Szyf, 2012; Brandes, 2008; Brown, Lipscomb, and Snyder,

2001). Those individuals who have antibodies against an antigen associated with a particular infectious disease will not be susceptible, even if they did not produce the antibody themselves (Purevdawa, Moon, Baigalmaa, Davaajav, Smith, and Vermund, 1997; Ramesh, Malla, Raju, Sehgal, Ganguly, Mahajan, and Dilawari, 1990). Examples of this phenomena include infants younger than six months who still have maternal antibodies passed through the placenta and from the colostrum, and adults who have had a recent injection of antibodies (Bausch and Schwarz, 2014; Bausch et al., 2001; Benner, Carabin, Sánchez-Serrano, Budke, and Carmena, 2010). However, these individuals soon return to the susceptible state as the antibodies are broken down (Rogers, Carolin, Vaught, and Compton, 2011; Ronohardjo and Rastiko, 1982; Sachs, 2001; Sachs and Malaney, 2002).

Some individuals may have a natural resistance to a particular infectious disease (Oleś, Gudowska-Nowak, and Kleczkowski, 2012; Otte, Nugent, and McLeod, 2004; Ozawa, Portnoy, Getaneh, Clark, Knoll, Bishai, and Patwardhan, 2016). However, except in some special cases such as malaria, these individuals make up such a small proportion of the total population that they can be ignored for the purposes of modeling an epidemic (Eaton and Groopman, 2013; Eckelman, Sherman, and MacNeill, 2018; Egger, 2011; Elbe, 2007; Ernst and Hay, 1994). Mathematical model of susceptibility is increasingly important when developing resilience measures (Moné, Ibikounlé, Massougbodji, and Mouahid, 2010; Morand, 2004; Moro, Budke, Schantz, Vasquez, Santivanez, and Villavicencio, 2011). The proportion of the population who are susceptible to a particular disease is denoted S (Foxman, 2002; Garner, Whan, Gard, and Phillips, 2001; Gayle and Hill, 2001; Gottstein, Pozio, and Nöckler, 2009). Due to the problems mentioned above, it is difficult to know this parameter for a given population (Hart and Halden, 2020; Häsler, Howe, and Stärk, 2011; Henschke, Kamper, and Maher, 2015; Hochberg, 1992). The advantage of estimating S in this way is that both the average age of infection and average life expectancy will be well documented, and thus the other parameters needed to calculate S will be easily at hand (Markos and Abdela, 2016; Martin and Shepherd, 2009; McGuinness, McGlynn, Johnson, MacIntyre, Batty, Burns, and McGinty, 2012).

Susceptibility in virology is critical because viruses are only able to cause disease or pathologies if they meet several criteria (Raut, 2004; Rehm, Mathers, Popova, Thavorncharoensap, Teerawattananon, and Patra, 2009; Rich and Perry, 2011). First, the virus is able to enter the cell, which is called a susceptible state. Second, there is a sufficient number of viruses within the cell (Howe, Häsler, and Stärk, 2013; Howe et al., 2012). Third, the virus is able to replicate within the cell which is called a permissive state (Arredondo and Zúñiga, 2006; Backer, van Roermund, Fischer, van Asseldonk, and Bergevoet, 2015; Bartsch, Hotez, Hertenstein, Diemert, Zapf, Bottazzi, and Lee, 2016). Hence susceptibility only refers to the fact that the virus is able to get into the cell, via having the proper receptors (Bergevoet, Van Schaik, Veling, Backus, and Franken, 2009; Binder, 1988; Bolos, Bacarea, and Marusteri, 2011). As a result, despite the fact that a host may be susceptible, the virus may still not be able to cause any pathologies within the host (Suhrcke, Stuckler, Suk, Desai, Senek, McKee, and Rechel, 2011; Šumilo, Bormane, Asokliene, Vasilenko, Golovljova, Avsic□Zupanc, and Randolph, 2008). Reasons for this are varied and may include suppression by the host immune system, or abortive measures taken by intrinsic cell defenses (Poundstone, Strathdee, and Celentano, 2004; Pritchett, Thilmany, and Johnson, 2005; Pugliatti, Beghi, Forsgren, Ekman, and Sobocki, 2007). Host tropism is the infection specificity of certain pathogens to particular hosts and host tissues (Armelagos, Brown, and Turner, 2005; Arokiasamy and Krishnan, 1994; Arora, 2001, 2005; Arredondo and Zúñiga, 2004). This type of tropism explains why most pathogens are only capable of infecting a limited range of host organisms (Krieger, 2001a, b; Lemma, 1969; Liu, Maniadakis, Gray, and Rayner, 2002; López, Torné, Franco, San-Martin, Viayna, Barrull, and Perulero, 2018).

Researchers can classify pathogenic organisms by the range of species and cell types that they exhibit host tropism for (Amuna and Zotor, 2008; Aral, Holmes, Padian, and Cates, 1996; Arbabi, Nezami, Hooshyar, and Delavari, 2018). For instance, pathogens that are able to infect a wide range of hosts and tissues are said to be amphotropic (Acemoglu and Johnson, 2007; Adda, 2016; Alloul, Sauriol, Kennedy, Laurier, Tessier, Novosel, and Contandriopoulos, 1998). Ecotropic pathogens, on the other hand, are only capable of infecting a narrow range of hosts and host tissue (St George, 1986; Steben and Duarte-Franco, 2007; Stehr-Green and Schantz, 1987; Stuckler, 2008; Stuckler and Siegel, 2011). Knowledge of a pathogen's host specificity allows professionals in the research and medical industries to model pathogenesis and develop vaccines, medication, and preventive measures to fight against infection (Uusküla, Müürsepp, Kawai, Raag, Jürisson, and Pillsbury, 2013; Vanni, Karnon, Madan, White, Edmunds, Foss, and Legood, 2011). Methods such as cell engineering, direct engineering and assisted evolution of host-adapted pathogens, and genome-wide genetic screens are currently being used by researchers to better understand the host range of a variety of different pathogenic organisms (Perry and Randolph, 1999; Philipson, 2000; Philipson and Posner, 1996; Pongchaiyakul, Songpattanasilp, and Taechakraichana, 2008). This chapter will close with an overview of community or herd immunity.

3.5. COMMUNITY IMMUNITY AND DECLINE IN FATALITIES

For purposes of this chapter, we have grouped together the last two phases of a disease epidemic as defined by the WHO. Phase 5 is characterized by human-to-human spread of the virus into at least two countries in one WHO regions (Weycker, Edelsberg, Oster, and Tino, 2005; Wu, Perrings, Kinzig, Collins, Minteer, and Daszak, 2017; Yach, Stuckler, and Brownell, 2006). While most countries will not be affected at this stage, the declaration of Phase 5 is a strong signal that a pandemic is imminent and that the time to finalize the organization, communication, and implementation of the planned mitigation measures is short (Chen, Li, Hsieh, Chang, Lee, Lee, and Ko, 2012; Conover, Pitt, Kessler, DuBow, and Sanborn, 1995; Crump, Murdoch, and Baker, 2001). Phase 6, the pandemic phase, is characterized by community-level outbreaks in at least one other country in a different WHO region in addition to the criteria defined in Phase 5 (Kim and Goldie, 2008; Klein, Laxminarayan, Smith, and Gilligan, 2007; Klepac, Laxminarayan, and Grenfell, 2011). Designation of this phase will indicate that a global pandemic is underway (Figure 3.5) (Abegunde and Stanciole, 2008; Abramowitz, Lacau Saint Guily, Moyal-Barracco, Bergeron, Borne, Dahlab, and Bénard, 2018).

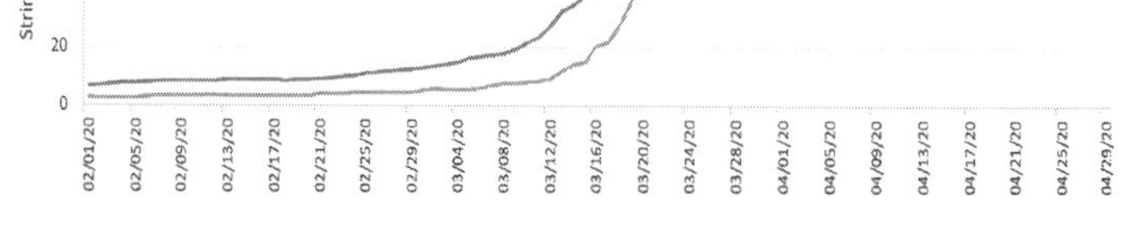

Figure 3.5. Government response in developing and developed nations to COVID-19.

Source: The United Nations.

During the post-peak period, pandemic disease levels in most countries with adequate surveillance will have dropped below peak observed levels (Jenkins, Baingana, Ahmad, McDaid, and Atun, 2011; Johnson, Alvarez-Pasquin, Bijl, Franco, Gaillat, Clara, and Weinke, 2015). The post-peak period signifies that pandemic activity appears to be decreasing; however, it is uncertain if additional waves will occur and countries will need to be prepared for a second wave (Pal, Kerorsa, Marami, and Kandi, 2020; Paterson, Otte, Slingenbergh, Wint, and Rogers, 2000; Pearce and Merletti, 2006). Previous pandemics have been characterized by waves of activity spread over months (Yi-Xin and Manderson, 2005; Zadoks, 2008; Zhan, Li, Wang, Sun, Geng, Xiong, and de Hoog, 2015; Zhang, Song, Cai, and Zhou, 2008). Once the level of disease activity drops, a critical communications task will be to balance this information with the possibility of another wave (Bwire, Munier, Ouedraogo, Heyerdahl, Komakech, Kagirita, and Makumbi, 2017; Canali, Aragrande, Angheben, Capelli, Drigo, Gobbi, and Cassini, 2020). Pandemic waves can be separated by months and an immediate "at-ease" signal may be premature (Buckley, 1984; Budke, Jiamin, Qian, and Torgerson, 2005; Bundy, Arámbulo III, and Grey, 1983; Buzby and Roberts, 2009). In the post-pandemic period, influenza disease activity will have returned to levels normally seen for seasonal influenza (Espinoza, Terashima, Herrera-Velit, and Marcos, 2010; Ezzati, Vander Hoorn, Lawes, Leach, James, Lopez, and Murray, 2005). It is expected that the pandemic virus will behave as a seasonal influenza A virus (Bonds, Keenan, Rohani, and Sachs, 2010; Boni, Galvani, Wickelgren, and Malani, 2013; Bonovas and Nikolopoulos, 2012). At this stage, it is important to maintain surveillance and update pandemic preparedness and response plans accordingly (Ozmen, Kurşun, and Ozcelik, 2005; Paarlberg, Hillberg, Lee, and Mathews, 2008; Paisley, Vraa-Andersen, Dybkjaer, Møller, Christensen, Mousing, and Agger, 1993). An intensive phase of recovery and evaluation may be required (Casamassimo, Thikkurissy, Edelstein, and Maiorini, 2009; Castro, Wilson, and Bloom, 2017).

Herd immunity (also called herd effect, community immunity, population immunity, or social immunity) is a form of indirect protection from infectious disease that occurs when a sufficient percentage of a population has become immune to an infection (St George, 1986; Steben and Duarte-Franco, 2007; Stehr-Green and Schantz, 1987; Stuckler, 2008; Stuckler and Siegel, 2011). This can occur through vaccination or previous infections, thereby reducing the likelihood of infection for individuals who lack immunity (Kim and Goldie, 2008; Klein, Laxminarayan, Smith, and Gilligan, 2007; Klepac,

Laxminarayan, and Grenfell, 2011). Immune individuals are unlikely to contribute to disease transmission, disrupting chains of infection, which stops or slows the spread of disease (Bonds, Keenan, Rohani, and Sachs, 2010; Boni, Galvani, Wickelgren, and Malani, 2013; Bonovas and Nikolopoulos, 2012). The greater the proportion of immune individuals in a community, the smaller the probability that non-immune individuals will come into contact with an infectious individual (Oleś, Gudowska-Nowak, and Kleczkowski, 2012; Otte, Nugent, and McLeod, 2004; Ozawa, Portnoy, Getaneh, Clark, Knoll, Bishai, and Patwardhan, 2016). Individuals can become immune by recovering from an earlier infection or through vaccination (Armelagos, Brown, and Turner, 2005; Arokiasamy and Krishnan, 1994; Arora, 2001, 2005; Arredondo and Zúñiga, 2004). Some individuals cannot become immune because of medical conditions, such as an immunodeficiency or immunosuppression, and for this group, herd immunity is a crucial method of protection (Bwire, Munier, Ouedraogo, Heyerdahl, Komakech, Kagirita, and Makumbi, 2017; Canali, Aragrande, Angheben, Capelli, Drigo, Gobbi, and Cassini, 2020).

Once the herd immunity threshold has been reached, disease gradually disappears from a population (Borghol, Suderman, McArdle, Racine, Hallett, Pembrey, and Szyf, 2012; Brandes, 2008; Brown, Lipscomb, and Snyder, 2001). This elimination, if achieved worldwide, may result in the permanent reduction in the number of infections to zero, called eradication (Peckham, 2013; Perrings et al., 2002, 2014). Herd immunity created via vaccination contributed to the eventual eradication of smallpox in 1977 and has contributed to the reduction of other diseases (Amuna and Zotor, 2008; Aral, Holmes, Padian, and Cates, 1996; Arbabi, Nezami, Hooshyar, and Delavari, 2018). Herd immunity applies only to contagious disease, meaning that it is transmitted from one individual to another (Acemoglu and Johnson, 2007; Adda, 2016; Alloul, Sauriol, Kennedy, Laurier, Tessier, Novosel, and Contandriopoulos, 1998). Tetanus, for example, is infectious but not contagious, so herd immunity does not apply (Eaton and Groopman, 2013; Eckelman, Sherman, and MacNeill, 2018; Egger, 2011; Elbe, 2007; Ernst and Hay, 1994).

Herd immunity was recognized as a naturally occurring phenomenon in the 1930s when it was observed that after a significant number of children had become immune to measles, the number of new infections temporarily decreased, including among the unvaccinated (Espinoza, Terashima, Herrera-Velit, and Marcos, 2010; Ezzati, Vander Hoorn, Lawes, Leach, James, Lopez, and Murray, 2005). Mass vaccination to induce herd immunity has since become common and proved successful in preventing the spread of many infectious diseases (Markos and Abdela, 2016; Martin and Shepherd, 2009; McGuinness, McGlynn, Johnson, MacIntyre, Batty, Burns, and McGinty, 2012). Opposition to vaccination has posed a challenge to herd immunity, allowing preventable diseases to persist in or return to populations with inadequate vaccination rates (Suhrcke, Stuckler, Suk, Desai, Senek, McKee, and Rechel, 2011; Šumilo, Bormane, Asokliene, Vasilenko, Golovljova, Avsic-Zupanc, and Randolph, 2008).

CHAPTER 3 SUMMARY

This chapter has explored the progress of a disease epidemic. Some of the stages that have been highlighted include origin or inception, spread, virulence, colonization of novel locations, changes in host characteristics, community immunity, and decline in case of fatalities. Obviously, these classifications are based on the generalized guidelines that are provided by the WHO. The guidance should not be taken as a template for future pandemics, since there are many examples of disease outbreaks taking slightly different patterns or even skipping some of the steps. In the next chapter, we consider the typologies of disease epidemics.

Chapter 4

Typologies of Disease Epidemics

CONTENTS

Many epidemic and pandemic typologies have arisen over time. Many of these emanate from a desire to understand the progress and impact of the outbreak so that lessons can be learned to be applied to future similar incidences. This chapter considers five major classifications based on the underlying cause, the populations affected, mode of transmission, an era in which they occurred, and the level of severity. By the end of this chapter, the reader should have a broad understanding of the implications of these classifications as well as their rationale.

4.1. CLASSIFICATION OF DISEASE EPIDEMICS BY THE UNDERLYING CAUSE

A disease is a particular abnormal condition that negatively affects the structure or function of all or part of an organism, and that is not due to any immediate external injury (Bergevoet, Van Schaik, Veling, Backus, and Franken, 2009; Binder, 1988; Bolos, Bacarea, and Marusteri, 2011). Diseases are often known to be medical conditions that are associated with specific symptoms and signs (Tapia, 2003; Torgerson and Dowling, 2001; Torgerson, Carmona, and Bonifacino, 2000; Uddin Khan, Atanasova, Krueger, Ramirez, and Gray, 2013). A disease may be caused by external factors such as pathogens or by internal dysfunctions (Moné, Ibikounlé, Massougbodji, and Mouahid, 2010; Morand, 2004; Moro, Budke, Schantz, Vasquez, Santivanez, and Villavicencio, 2011). For example, internal dysfunctions of the immune system can produce a variety of different diseases, including various forms of immunodeficiency, hypersensitivity, allergies, and autoimmune disorders (Uusküla, Müürsepp, Kawai, Raag, Jürisson, and Pillsbury, 2013; Vanni, Karnon, Madan, White, Edmunds, Foss, and Legood, 2011). Regardless of their classification, disease epidemics tend to mostly affect the poorest living in the poorest community (Raut, 2004; Rehm, Mathers, Popova, Thavorncharoensap, Teerawattananon, and Patra, 2009; Rich and Perry, 2011). In the case of COVID-19, the highest deaths are surprisingly in the developed world (Foxman, 2002; Garner, Whan, Gard, and Phillips, 2001; Gayle and Hill, 2001; Gottstein, Pozio, and Nöckler, 2009). However, there are signs that there will be numerous channels through which the wider economic impact will reach the developing world (see Figure 4.1).

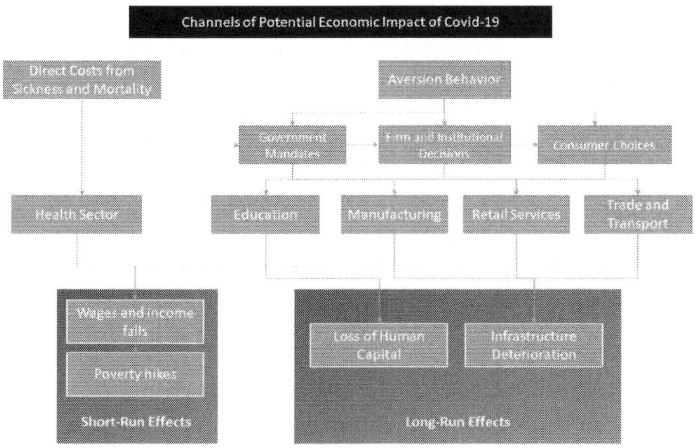

Figure 4.1. Impact of COVID-19 on low- and middle-income countries.

Source: Center for Global Development.

In humans, disease is often used more broadly to refer to any condition that causes pain, dysfunction, distress, social problems, or death to the person afflicted, or similar problems for those in contact with the person (Howe, Häsler, and Stärk, 2013; Howe et al., 2012). In this broader sense, it sometimes includes injuries, disabilities, disorders, syndromes, infections, isolated symptoms, deviant behaviors, and atypical variations of structure and function, while in other contexts and for other purposes these may be considered distinguishable categories (Weycker, Edelsberg, Oster, and Tino, 2005; Wu, Perrings, Kinzig, Collins, Minteer, and Daszak, 2017; Yach, Stuckler, and Brownell, 2006). Diseases can affect people not only physically, but also mentally, as contracting and living with a disease can alter the affected person's perspective on life (Daily, and Ehrlich, 1996; Deogaonkar, Hutubessy, Van Der Putten, Evers, and Jit, 2012; Dorn, 1992; Ducrotoy, Bertu, Ocholi, Gusi, Bryssinckx, Welburn, and Moriyon, 2014).

Death due to disease is called death by natural causes. There are four main types of disease: infectious diseases, deficiency diseases, hereditary diseases (including both genetic diseases and non-genetic hereditary diseases), and physiological diseases (Chen, Li, Hsieh, Chang, Lee, Lee, and Ko, 2012; Conover, Pitt, Kessler, DuBow, and Sanborn, 1995; Crump, Murdoch, and Baker, 2001). Diseases can also be classified in other ways, such as communicable versus non-communicable diseases (Arredondo and Zúñiga, 2006; Backer, van Roermund, Fischer, van Asseldonk, and Bergevoet, 2015; Bartsch, Hotez, Hertenstein, Diemert, Zapf, Bottazzi, and Lee, 2016). The deadliest diseases in humans are coronary artery disease (blood flow obstruction), followed by cerebrovascular disease and lower respiratory infections (Rogers, Carolin, Vaught, and Compton, 2011; Ronohardjo and Rastiko, 1982; Sachs, 2001; Sachs and Malaney, 2002). In developed countries, the diseases that cause the vast majority of cases of sickness overall are neuropsychiatric conditions, such as depression and anxiety (Yi-Xin and Manderson, 2005; Zadoks, 2008; Zhan, Li, Wang, Sun, Geng, Xiong, and de Hoog, 2015; Zhang, Song, Cai, and Zhou, 2008). The study of disease is called pathology, which includes the study of etiology, or cause (Perry and Randolph, 1999; Philipson, 2000; Philipson and Posner, 1996; Pongchaiyakul, Songpattanasilp, and Taechakraichana, 2008). In many cases, terms such as disease, disorder, morbidity, sickness, and illness are used interchangeably (Abegunde and Stanciole, 2008; Abramowitz, Lacau Saint Guily, Moyal-Barracco, Bergeron, Borne, Dahlab, and Bénard, 2018). However, there are situations when specific terms are considered preferable (Fenichel, 2013; Fenichel et al., 2011; Fogel, 1994).

The term disease broadly refers to any condition that impairs the normal functioning of the body (Saleha, 1991; Sibert, Rigaud, Delavierre, and Labat, 2010; Skrepnek and Skrepnek, 2004; Sloane, 2009; Sockett, 1993). For this reason, diseases are associated with dysfunction of the body's normal homeostatic processes (Bausch and Schwarz, 2014; Bausch et al., 2001; Benner, Carabin, Sánchez-Serrano, Budke, and Carmena, 2010). Commonly, the term is used to refer specifically to infectious diseases, which are clinically evident diseases that result from the presence of pathogenic microbial agents, including viruses, bacteria, fungi, protozoa, multicellular organisms, and aberrant proteins known as prions (Hart and Halden, 2020; Häsler, Howe, and Stärk, 2011; Henschke, Kamper, and Maher, 2015; Hochberg, 1992). An infection or colonization that does not and will not produce clinically evident impairment of normal functioning, such as the presence of the normal bacteria and yeasts in the gut, or of a passenger virus, is not considered a disease (Ozmen, Kurşun, and Ozcelik, 2005; Paarlberg, Hillberg, Lee, and Mathews, 2008; Paisley, Vraa-Andersen, Dybkjaer, Møller, Christensen, Mousing, and Agger, 1993). By contrast, an infection that is asymptomatic during its incubation period, but expected to produce symptoms later, is usually considered a disease (Buckley, 1984; Budke, Jiamin, Qian, and Torgerson, 2005; Bundy, Arámbulo III, and Grey, 1983; Buzby and Roberts, 2009). Non-infectious diseases are all other diseases, including most forms of cancer, heart disease, and genetic disease (Pal, Kerorsa, Marami, and Kandi, 2020; Paterson, Otte, Slingenbergh, Wint, and Rogers, 2000; Pearce and Merletti, 2006). An acquired disease is one that began at some point during one's lifetime, as opposed to disease that was already present at birth, which is congenital disease (Narrod, Zinsstag, and Tiongco, 2012; Nascimento and de Oliveira, 2014; O'Brien, Lahue, Caro, and Davidson, 2007). Acquired sounds like it could mean "caught via contagion," but it simply means acquired sometime after birth (Krieger, 2001a, b; Lemma, 1969; Liu, Maniadakis, Gray, and Rayner, 2002; López, Torné, Franco, San-Martin, Viayna, Barrull, and Perulero, 2018). It also sounds like it could imply secondary disease, but acquired disease can be primary disease (Jenkins, Baingana, Ahmad, McDaid, and Atun, 2011; Johnson, Alvarez-Pasquin, Bijl, Franco, Gaillat, Clara, and Weinke, 2015). An acute disease is one of a short-term nature (acute); the term sometimes also connotes a fulminant nature (Purevdawa, Moon, Baigalmaa, Davaajav, Smith, and Vermund, 1997; Ramesh, Malla, Raju, Sehgal, Ganguly, Mahajan, and Dilawari, 1990). A chronic disease is one that persists over time, often characterized as at least six months but may also include illnesses that are expected to last for the entirety of one's natural life (Jenkins, Baingana, Ahmad, McDaid, and Atun, 2011; Johnson, Alvarez-Pasquin, Bijl, Franco, Gaillat, Clara, and Weinke, 2015). A congenital disorder is one that is present at birth (Krieger, 2001a, b; Lemma, 1969; Liu, Maniadakis, Gray, and Rayner, 2002; López, Torné, Franco, San-Martin, Viayna, Barrull, and Perulero, 2018). It is often a genetic disease or disorder and can be inherited (Narrod, Zinsstag, and Tiongco, 2012; Nascimento and de Oliveira, 2014; O'Brien, Lahue, Caro, and Davidson, 2007). This can also be the result of a vertically transmitted infection from the mother, such as HIV/AIDS (Pal, Kerorsa, Marami, and Kandi, 2020; Paterson, Otte, Slingenbergh, Wint, and Rogers, 2000; Pearce and Merletti, 2006).

A genetic disorder or disease is caused by one or more genetic mutations (Buckley, 1984; Budke, Jiamin, Qian, and Torgerson, 2005; Bundy, Arámbulo III, and Grey, 1983; Buzby and Roberts, 2009). It is often inherited, but some mutations are random and de novo (Ozmen, Kurşun, and Ozcelik, 2005; Paarlberg, Hillberg, Lee, and Mathews, 2008; Paisley, Vraa-Andersen, Dybkjaer, Møller, Christensen, Mousing, and Agger, 1993). A hereditary disease is a type of genetic disease caused by genetic mutations that are hereditary and can therefore run in families (Hart and Halden, 2020; Häsler, Howe, and Stärk, 2011; Henschke, Kamper, and Maher, 2015; Hochberg, 1992). An iatrogenic disease or condition is one that is caused by medical intervention, whether as a side effect of a treatment or as an inadvertent outcome (Bausch and Schwarz, 2014; Bausch et al., 2001; Benner, Carabin,

Sánchez-Serrano, Budke, and Carmena, 2010). An idiopathic disease has an unknown cause or source (Saleha, 1991; Sibert, Rigaud, Delavierre, and Labat, 2010; Skrepnek and Skrepnek, 2004; Sloane, 2009; Sockett, 1993). As medical science has advanced, many diseases with entirely unknown causes have had some aspects of their sources explained and therefore shed their idiopathic status (Fenichel, 2013; Fenichel et al., 2011; Fogel, 1994). For example, when germs were discovered, it became known that they were a cause of infection, but particular germs and diseases had not been linked (Abegunde and Stanciole, 2008; Abramowitz, Lacau Saint Guily, Moyal-Barracco, Bergeron, Borne, Dahlab, and Bénard, 2018). Incurable diseases are not necessarily terminal diseases, and sometimes a disease's symptoms can be treated sufficiently for the disease to have little or no impact on quality of life (Perry and Randolph, 1999; Philipson, 2000; Philipson and Posner, 1996; Pongchaiyakul, Songpattanasilp, and Taechakraichana, 2008).

A primary disease is a disease that is due to a root cause of illness, as opposed to secondary disease, which is a sequela, or complication that is caused by the primary disease (Yi-Xin and Manderson, 2005; Zadoks, 2008; Zhan, Li, Wang, Sun, Geng, Xiong, and de Hoog, 2015; Zhang, Song, Cai, and Zhou, 2008). For example, a common cold is a primary disease, where rhinitis is a possible secondary disease, or sequela (Rogers, Carolin, Vaught, and Compton, 2011; Ronohardjo and Rastiko, 1982; Sachs, 2001; Sachs and Malaney, 2002). A doctor must determine what primary disease, a cold or bacterial infection, is causing a patient's secondary rhinitis when deciding whether or not to prescribe antibiotics (Arredondo and Zúñiga, 2006; Backer, van Roermund, Fischer, van Asseldonk, and Bergevoet, 2015; Bartsch, Hotez, Hertenstein, Diemert, Zapf, Bottazzi, and Lee, 2016). A secondary disease is a disease that is a sequela or complication of a prior, causal disease, which is referred to as the primary disease or simply the underlying cause or root cause (Chen, Li, Hsieh, Chang, Lee, Lee, and Ko, 2012; Conover, Pitt, Kessler, DuBow, and Sanborn, 1995; Crump, Murdoch, and Baker, 2001). For example, a bacterial infection can be primary, wherein a healthy person is exposed to a bacteria and becomes infected, or it can be secondary to a primary cause, that predisposes the body to infection (Daily, and Ehrlich, 1996; Deogaonkar, Hutubessy, Van Der Putten, Evers, and Jit, 2012; Dorn, 1992; Ducrotoy, Bertu, Ocholi, Gusi, Bryssinckx, Welburn, and Moriyon, 2014). In the next section, we consider the classification of diseases by the populations that they mostly affect.

4.2. CLASSIFICATION OF DISEASE EPIDEMICS BY THE POPULATIONS AFFECTED

Recently, there was disquiet about how some powerful politicians were seeking to localize the COVID-19 outbreak by giving it names that were tinged with hints of racism and xenophobia. There is a long history of disease classification that is meant to implicitly assign blame for its outbreak (Weycker, Edelsberg, Oster, and Tino, 2005; Wu, Perrings, Kinzig, Collins, Minteer, and Daszak, 2017; Yach, Stuckler, and Brownell, 2006). Hence, the Spanish flue becomes innately "Spanish" and the "Great Plagues of London" are urbanized (Howe, Häsler, and Stärk, 2013; Howe et al., 2012). Although this is a social phenomenon that reflects the prejudices of a community, there is a scientific basis for linking disease epidemicsDisease epidemics to particular geographical locations (Foxman, 2002; Garner, Whan, Gard, and Phillips, 2001; Gayle and Hill, 2001; Gottstein, Pozio, and Nöckler, 2009). This is particularly appropriate if that epidemic has not shifted away from a particular area or if it is markedly different from similar epidemics in another area (Raut, 2004; Rehm, Mathers, Popova, Thavorncharoensap, Teerawattananon, and Patra, 2009; Rich and Perry, 2011). Of course, the classification may lose relevance if the outbreak spreads widely and the strains become closer to each other in terms of their characteristics (Uusküla, Müürsepp, Kawai, Raag, Jürisson, and Pillsbury, 2013; Vanni, Karnon, Madan, White, Edmunds, Foss, and Legood, 2011). The geographical mapping of disease epidemicscan also assist in learning about the impact of response police, a case in point being social distancing in the Spanish Flue and COVID-19 crises (see Figure 4.2).

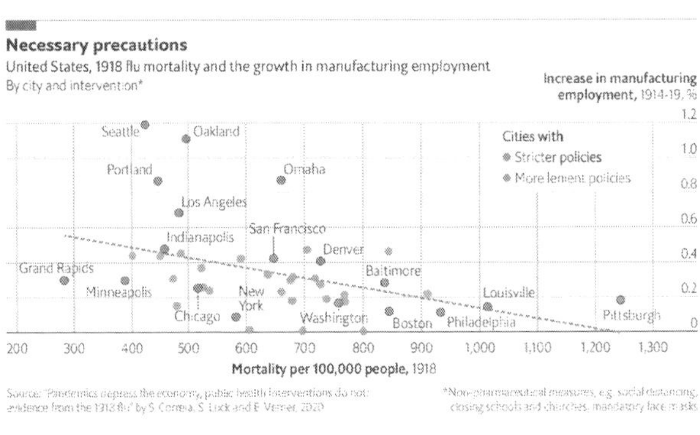

Figure 4.2. Lessons from the Spanish flue and social distancing.

Source: The Economist.

Epidemiology is the study of the factors that cause or encourage diseases (Moné, Ibikounlé, Massougbodji, and Mouahid, 2010; Morand, 2004; Moro, Budke, Schantz, Vasquez, Santivanez, and Villavicencio, 2011). Some diseases are more common in certain geographic areas, among people with certain genetic or socioeconomic characteristics, or at different times of the year (Tapia, 2003; Torgerson and Dowling, 2001; Torgerson, Carmona, and Bonifacino, 2000; Uddin Khan, Atanasova, Krueger, Ramirez, and Gray, 2013). Epidemiology is considered a cornerstone methodology of public health research and is highly regarded in evidence-based medicine for identifying risk factors for diseases (Bergevoet, Van Schaik, Veling, Backus, and Franken, 2009; Binder, 1988; Bolos, Bacarea, and Marusteri, 2011). In the study of communicable and non-communicable diseases, the work of epidemiologists ranges from outbreak investigation to study design, data collection, and analysis (Suhrcke, Stuckler, Suk, Desai, Senek, McKee, and Rechel, 2011; Šumilo, Bormane, Asokliene, Vasilenko, Golovljova, Avsic-Zupanc, and Randolph, 2008). This necessarily includes the development of statistical models to test hypotheses and the documentation of results for submission to peer-reviewed journals (Markos and Abdela, 2016; Martin and Shepherd, 2009; McGuinness, McGlynn, Johnson, MacIntyre, Batty, Burns, and McGinty, 2012).

Epidemiologists also study the interaction of diseases in a population, a condition known as a syndemic (Espinoza, Terashima, Herrera-Velit, and Marcos, 2010; Ezzati, Vander Hoorn, Lawes, Leach, James, Lopez, and Murray, 2005). Epidemiologists rely on a number of other scientific disciplines (Eaton and Groopman, 2013; Eckelman, Sherman, and MacNeill, 2018; Egger, 2011; Elbe, 2007; Ernst and Hay, 1994). For example, biology helps them to better understand disease processes (Acemoglu and Johnson, 2007; Adda, 2016; Alloul, Sauriol, Kennedy, Laurier, Tessier, Novosel, and Contandriopoulos, 1998). They use biostatistics to analyze and utilize the current raw information available (Amuna and Zotor, 2008; Aral, Holmes, Padian, and Cates, 1996; Arbabi, Nezami, Hooshyar, and Delavari, 2018). Others may refer to geographic information science in order to store data and map disease patterns (Peckham, 2013; Perrings et al., 2002, 2014). Additionally, the social science disciplines help them to better understand proximate and distal risk factors (Borghol, Suderman, McArdle, Racine, Hallett, Pembrey, and Szyf, 2012; Brandes, 2008; Brown, Lipscomb, and Snyder, 2001). Epidemiology can help identify causes as well as guide prevention efforts. In studying diseases, epidemiology faces the challenge of defining them (Bwire, Munier, Ouedraogo, Heyerdahl, Komakech, Kagirita, and Makumbi, 2017; Canali, Aragrande, Angheben, Capelli, Drigo, Gobbi, and Cassini, 2020). Especially for poorly understood diseases, different groups might use significantly different definitions (Armelagos, Brown, and Turner, 2005; Arokiasamy and Krishnan, 1994; Arora, 2001, 2005; Arredondo and Zúñiga, 2004). Without an agreed-on definition, different researchers may report different numbers of cases and characteristics of the disease (Oleś, Gudowska-Nowak, and Kleczkowski, 2012; Otte, Nugent, and McLeod, 2004; Ozawa, Portnoy, Getaneh, Clark, Knoll, Bishai, and Patwardhan, 2016).

Some morbidity databases are compiled with data supplied by states and territories health authorities, at national levels or larger scale, such as is the case with the European Hospital Morbidity Database (Bonds, Keenan, Rohani, and Sachs, 2010; Boni, Galvani, Wickelgren, and Malani, 2013; Bonovas and Nikolopoulos, 2012). This is a significant database that services the European Union and which may contain hospital discharge data by detailed diagnosis, age, and sex (Kim and Goldie, 2008; Klein, Laxminarayan, Smith, and Gilligan, 2007; Klepac, Laxminarayan, and Grenfell, 2011). The European HMDB data was submitted by European countries to the World Health Organization (WHO) Regional Office for Europe (St George, 1986; Steben and Duarte-Franco, 2007; Stehr-Green and Schantz, 1987; Stuckler, 2008; Stuckler and Siegel, 2011). Disease burden is the impact of a health problem in an area measured by financial cost, mortality, morbidity, or other indicators (Poundstone, Strathdee, and Celentano, 2004; Pritchett, Thilmany, and Johnson, 2005; Pugliatti, Beghi, Forsgren, Ekman, and Sobocki, 2007). There are several measures used to quantify the burden imposed by diseases on people (Casamassimo, Thikkurissy, Edelstein, and Maiorini, 2009; Castro, Wilson, and Bloom, 2017). The years of potential life lost (YPLL) is a simple estimate of the number of years that a person's life was shortened due to a disease (Yi-Xin and Manderson, 2005; Zadoks, 2008; Zhan, Li, Wang, Sun, Geng, Xiong, and de Hoog, 2015; Zhang, Song, Cai, and Zhou, 2008). For example, if a person dies at the age of 55 from a disease, and would probably have lived until age 75 without that disease, then that disease has caused a loss of 20 years of potential life (Weycker, Edelsberg, Oster, and Tino, 2005; Wu, Perrings, Kinzig, Collins, Minteer, and Daszak, 2017; Yach, Stuckler, and Brownell, 2006). YPLL measurements do not account for how disabled a person is before dying (Uusküla, Müürsepp, Kawai, Raag, Jürisson, and Pillsbury, 2013; Vanni, Karnon, Madan, White, Edmunds, Foss, and Legood, 2011). Hence, the measurement treats a person who dies suddenly and a person who died at the same age after decades of illness as equivalent (Tapia, 2003; Torgerson and Dowling, 2001; Torgerson, Carmona, and Bonifacino, 2000; Uddin Khan, Atanasova, Krueger, Ramirez, and Gray, 2013). In 2004, the WHO calculated that 932 million years of potential life were lost to premature death (Suhrcke, Stuckler, Suk, Desai, Senek, McKee, and Rechel, 2011; Šumilo, Bormane, Asokliene, Vasilenko, Golovljova, Avsic-Zupanc, and Randolph, 2008).

The quality-adjusted life-year (QALY) and disability-adjusted life year (DALY) metrics are similar but take into account whether the person was healthy after diagnosis (St George, 1986; Steben and Duarte-Franco, 2007; Stehr-Green and Schantz, 1987; Stuckler, 2008; Stuckler and Siegel, 2011). In addition to the number of years lost due to premature death, these measurements add part of the years lost to being sick (Saleha, 1991; Sibert, Rigaud, Delavierre, and Labat, 2010; Skrepnek and Skrepnek, 2004; Sloane, 2009; Sockett, 1993). Unlike YPLL, these measurements show the burden imposed on people who are very sick, but who live a normal lifespan (Rogers, Carolin, Vaught, and Compton, 2011; Ronohardjo and Rastiko, 1982; Sachs, 2001; Sachs and Malaney, 2002). A disease that has high morbidity, but low mortality, has a high DALY and a low YPLL (Raut, 2004; Rehm, Mathers, Popova, Thavorncharoensap, Teerawattananon, and Patra, 2009; Rich and Perry, 2011). In 2004, the WHO calculated that 1.5 billion DALYs were lost to disease and injury (Purevdawa, Moon, Baigalmaa, Davaajav, Smith, and Vermund, 1997; Ramesh, Malla, Raju, Sehgal, Ganguly, Mahajan, and Dilawari, 1990). In the developed world, heart disease and stroke cause the most loss of life, but neuropsychiatric conditions like major depressive disorder cause the most years lost to being sick (Poundstone, Strathdee, and Celentano, 2004; Pritchett, Thilmany, and Johnson, 2005; Pugliatti, Beghi, Forsgren, Ekman, and Sobocki, 2007).

The ways in which a society responds to diseases is the subject of medical sociology and increased public interest (Perry and Randolph, 1999; Philipson, 2000; Philipson and Posner, 1996; Pongchaiyakul, Songpattanasilp, and Taechakraichana, 2008). This is particularly true if there are significant diversities in the local responses (Peckham, 2013; Perrings et al., 2002, 2014). A condition may be considered a disease in some cultures or eras but not in others (Pal, Kerorsa, Marami, and Kandi, 2020; Paterson, Otte, Slingenbergh, Wint, and Rogers, 2000; Pearce and Merletti, 2006). For example, obesity can represent wealth and abundance, and is a status symbol in famine-prone areas and some places hard-hit by HIV/AIDS (Ozmen, Kurşun, and Ozcelik, 2005; Paarlberg, Hillberg, Lee, and Mathews,

2008; Paisley, Vraa-Andersen, Dybkjaer, Møller, Christensen, Mousing, and Agger, 1993). Epilepsy is considered a sign of spiritual gifts among the Hmong people (Oleś, Gudowska-Nowak, and Kleczkowski, 2012; Otte, Nugent, and McLeod, 2004; Ozawa, Portnoy, Getaneh, Clark, Knoll, Bishai, and Patwardhan, 2016). Sickness confers the social legitimization of certain benefits, such as illness benefits, work avoidance, and being looked after by others (Narrod, Zinsstag, and Tiongco, 2012; Nascimento and de Oliveira, 2014; O'Brien, Lahue, Caro, and Davidson, 2007). The person who is sick takes on a social role called the sick role (Moné, Ibikounlé, Massougbodji, and Mouahid, 2010; Morand, 2004; Moro, Budke, Schantz, Vasquez, Santivanez, and Villavicencio, 2011). A person who responds to a dreaded disease, such as cancer, in a culturally acceptable fashion may be publicly and privately honored with higher social status (Markos and Abdela, 2016; Martin and Shepherd, 2009; McGuinness, McGlynn, Johnson, MacIntyre, Batty, Burns, and McGinty, 2012). In return for these benefits, the sick person is obligated to seek treatment and work to become well once more (Krieger, 2001a, b; Lemma, 1969; Liu, Maniadakis, Gray, and Rayner, 2002; López, Torné, Franco, San-Martin, Viayna, Barrull, and Perulero, 2018). As a comparison, consider pregnancy, which is not interpreted as a disease or sickness, even if the mother and baby may both benefit from medical care (Kim and Goldie, 2008; Klein, Laxminarayan, Smith, and Gilligan, 2007; Klepac, Laxminarayan, and Grenfell, 2011).

Most religions grant exceptions from religious duties to people who are sick (Jenkins, Baingana, Ahmad, McDaid, and Atun, 2011; Johnson, Alvarez-Pasquin, Bijl, Franco, Gaillat, Clara, and Weinke, 2015). For example, one whose life would be endangered by fasting on Yom Kippur or during Ramadan is exempted from the requirement, or even forbidden from participating (Howe, Häsler, and Stärk, 2013; Howe et al., 2012). People who are sick are also exempted from social duties (Hart and Halden, 2020; Häsler, Howe, and Stärk, 2011; Henschke, Kamper, and Maher, 2015; Hochberg, 1992). For example, ill-health is the only socially acceptable reason for an American to refuse an invitation to the White House (Foxman, 2002; Garner, Whan, Gard, and Phillips, 2001; Gayle and Hill, 2001; Gottstein, Pozio, and Nöckler, 2009). The identification of a condition as a disease, rather than as simply a variation of human structure or function, can have significant social or economic implications (Fenichel, 2013; Fenichel et al., 2011; Fogel, 1994). The controversial recognition of diseases such as repetitive stress injury (RSI) and post-traumatic stress disorder (PTSD) has had a number of positive and negative effects on the financial and other responsibilities of governments, corporations, and institutions towards individuals, as well as on the individuals themselves (Espinoza, Terashima, Herrera-Velit, and Marcos, 2010; Ezzati, Vander Hoorn, Lawes, Leach, James, Lopez, and Murray, 2005). The social implication of viewing aging as a disease could be profound, though this classification is not yet widespread (Eaton and Groopman, 2013; Eckelman, Sherman, and MacNeill, 2018; Egger, 2011; Elbe, 2007; Ernst and Hay, 1994).

Lepers were people who were historically shunned because they had an infectious disease, and the term "leper" still evokes social stigma (Daily, and Ehrlich, 1996; Deogaonkar, Hutubessy, Van Der Putten, Evers, and Jit, 2012; Dorn, 1992; Ducrotoy, Bertu, Ocholi, Gusi, Bryssinckx, Welburn, and Moriyon, 2014). Fear of disease can still be a widespread social phenomenon, though not all diseases evoke extreme social stigma (Chen, Li, Hsieh, Chang, Lee, Lee, and Ko, 2012; Conover, Pitt, Kessler, DuBow, and Sanborn, 1995; Crump, Murdoch, and Baker, 2001). Social standing and economic status affect health (Casamassimo, Thikkurissy, Edelstein, and Maiorini, 2009; Castro, Wilson, and Bloom, 2017). Diseases of poverty are diseases that are associated with poverty and low social status (Bwire, Munier, Ouedraogo, Heyerdahl, Komakech, Kagirita, and Makumbi, 2017; Canali, Aragrande, Angheben, Capelli, Drigo, Gobbi, and Cassini, 2020). However, diseases of affluence are diseases that are associated with high social and economic status (Buckley, 1984; Budke, Jiamin, Qian, and Torgerson, 2005; Bundy, Arámbulo III, and Grey, 1983; Buzby and Roberts, 2009); which diseases are associated with which states vary according to time, place, and technology (Borghol, Suderman, McArdle, Racine, Hallett, Pembrey, and Szyf, 2012; Brandes, 2008; Brown, Lipscomb, and Snyder, 2001). Some diseases, such as diabetes mellitus, may be associated with both poverty (poor food choices) and affluence (long lifespans and sedentary lifestyles), through different mechanisms (Bonds, Keenan, Rohani, and Sachs, 2010; Boni, Galvani, Wickelgren, and Malani, 2013; Bonovas and Nikolopoulos, 2012). The term lifestyle diseases describe diseases associated with longevity and that are more common among older people (Bergevoet, Van Schaik, Veling, Backus, and Franken, 2009; Binder, 1988; Bolos, Bacarea, and Marusteri, 2011). For example, cancer is far more common in societies in which most members live until they reach the age of 80 than in societies in which most members die before they reach the age of 50 (Bausch and Schwarz, 2014; Bausch et al., 2001; Benner, Carabin, Sánchez-Serrano, Budke, and Carmena, 2010). The next section considers the classification of disease according to mode of transmission.

4.3. CLASSIFICATION OF DISEASE EPIDEMICS BY MODE OF TRANSMISSION

In medicine, public health, and biology, transmission is the passing of a pathogen causing communicable disease from an infected host individual or group to a particular individual or group (Arredondo and Zúñiga, 2006; Backer, van Roermund, Fischer, van Asseldonk, and Bergevoet, 2015; Bartsch, Hotez, Hertenstein, Diemert, Zapf, Bottazzi, and Lee, 2016). This occurs regardless of whether the other individual was previously infected (Armelagos, Brown, and Turner, 2005; Arokiasamy and Krishnan, 1994; Arora, 2001, 2005; Arredondo and Zúñiga, 2004). The term strictly refers to the transmission of microorganisms directly from one individual to another by one or more a given number of means (Amuna and Zotor, 2008; Aral, Holmes, Padian, and Cates, 1996; Arbabi, Nezami, Hooshyar, and Delavari, 2018). For example, airborne transmission occurs when very small dry and wet particles that stay in the air for long periods of time allowing airborne contamination even after the departure of the host (Figure 4.3) (Acemoglu and Johnson, 2007; Adda, 2016; Alloul, Sauriol, Kennedy, Laurier, Tessier, Novosel, and Contandriopoulos, 1998).

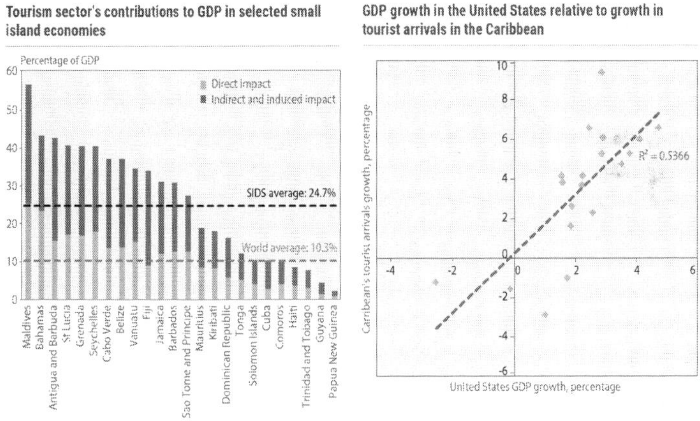

Figure 4.3. Challenges faced by small island developing nations during the COVID-19 pandemic.

Source: The United Nations.

In droplet transmission, small, and usually wet particles that stay in the air for a short period of time. Contamination usually occurs in the presence of the host (Abegunde and Stanciole, 2008; Abramowitz, Lacau Saint Guily,

Moyal-Barracco, Bergeron, Borne, Dahlab, and Bénard, 2018). Direct physical contact occurs when touching an infected individual, including sexual contact (Ozmen, Kurşun, and Ozcelik, 2005; Paarlberg, Hillberg, Lee, and Mathews, 2008; Paisley, Vraa-Andersen, Dybkjaer, Møller, Christensen, Mousing, and Agger, 1993). In indirect physical contact, transmission usually occurs by touching a contaminated surface, including soil or fomite (Bonds, Keenan, Rohani, and Sachs, 2010; Boni, Galvani, Wickelgren, and Malani, 2013; Bonovas and Nikolopoulos, 2012). During fecal-oral transmission, the modality is usually from unwashed hands, contaminated food or water sources due to lack of sanitation and hygiene (Espinoza, Terashima, Herrera-Velit, and Marcos, 2010; Ezzati, Vander Hoorn, Lawes, Leach, James, Lopez, and Murray, 2005). This is an important transmission route in pediatrics, veterinary medicine and developing countries (Buckley, 1984; Budke, Jiamin, Qian, and Torgerson, 2005; Bundy, Arámbulo III, and Grey, 1983; Buzby and Roberts, 2009).

Transmission can also be indirect, via another organism, either a vector (e.g., a mosquito or fly) or an intermediate host, such as the tapeworm in pigs which can be transmitted to humans who ingest improperly cooked pork (Bwire, Munier, Ouedraogo, Heyerdahl, Komakech, Kagirita, and Makumbi, 2017; Canali, Aragrande, Angheben, Capelli, Drigo, Gobbi, and Cassini, 2020). Indirect transmission could involve zoonoses or, more typically, larger pathogens like macroparasites with more complex life cycles (Yi-Xin and Manderson, 2005; Zadoks, 2008; Zhan, Li, Wang, Sun, Geng, Xiong, and de Hoog, 2015; Zhang, Song, Cai, and Zhou, 2008). Transmissions can be autochthonous (i.e., between two individuals in the same place) or may involve travel of the microorganism or the affected hosts (Pal, Kerorsa, Marami, and Kandi, 2020; Paterson, Otte, Slingenbergh, Wint, and Rogers, 2000; Pearce and Merletti, 2006). An infectious disease agent can be transmitted in two ways (Jenkins, Baingana, Ahmad, McDaid, and Atun, 2011; Johnson, Alvarez-Pasquin, Bijl, Franco, Gaillat, Clara, and Weinke, 2015). First, as horizontal disease agent transmission from one individual to another in the same generation who are peers in the same age group (Abegunde and Stanciole, 2008; Abramowitz, Lacau Saint Guily, Moyal-Barracco, Bergeron, Borne, Dahlab, and Bénard, 2018). The second category occurs by either direct contact (licking, touching, biting), or indirect contact through air via a cough or sneeze (Kim and Goldie, 2008; Klein, Laxminarayan, Smith, and Gilligan, 2007; Klepac, Laxminarayan, and Grenfell, 2011). This is because vectors or fomites that allow the transmission of the agent causing the disease without physical contact

(Chen, Li, Hsieh, Chang, Lee, Lee, and Ko, 2012; Conover, Pitt, Kessler, DuBow, and Sanborn, 1995; Crump, Murdoch, and Baker, 2001). Another modality is by vertical disease transmission, passing the agent causing the disease from parent to offspring, such as in prenatal or perinatal transmission (Weycker, Edelsberg, Oster, and Tino, 2005; Wu, Perrings, Kinzig, Collins, Minteer, and Daszak, 2017; Yach, Stuckler, and Brownell, 2006).

The term infectivity describes the ability of an organism to enter, survive, and multiply in the host, while the infectiousness of a disease agent indicates the comparative ease with which the disease agent is transmitted to other hosts (Perry and Randolph, 1999; Philipson, 2000; Philipson and Posner, 1996; Pongchaiyakul, Songpattanasilp, and Taechakraichana, 2008). Transmission of pathogen can occur in various ways including physical contact, contaminated food, body fluids, objects, airborne inhalation, or through vector organisms (Uusküla, Müürsepp, Kawai, Raag, Jürisson, and Pillsbury, 2013; Vanni, Karnon, Madan, White, Edmunds, Foss, and Legood, 2011). The term community transmission means that the source of infection for the spread of an illness is unknown or a link in terms of contacts between patients and other people is missing (St George, 1986; Steben and Duarte-Franco, 2007; Stehr-Green and Schantz, 1987; Stuckler, 2008; Stuckler and Siegel, 2011). It refers to the difficulty in grasping the epidemiological link in the community beyond confirmed cases (Acemoglu and Johnson, 2007; Adda, 2016; Alloul, Sauriol, Kennedy, Laurier, Tessier, Novosel, and Contandriopoulos, 1998). The term local transmission means that the source of the infection has been identified within the reporting location, such as within a country, region or city (Amuna and Zotor, 2008; Aral, Holmes, Padian, and Cates, 1996; Arbabi, Nezami, Hooshyar, and Delavari, 2018).

The route of transmission is important to epidemiologists because patterns of contact vary between different populations and different groups of populations depending on socio-economic, cultural, and other features (Krieger, 2001a, b; Lemma, 1969; Liu, Maniadakis, Gray, and Rayner, 2002; López, Torné, Franco, San-Martin, Viayna, Barrull, and Perulero, 2018). For example, low personal and food hygiene due to the lack of a clean water supply may result in increased transmission of diseases by the fecal-oral route, such as cholera (Armelagos, Brown, and Turner, 2005; Arokiasamy and Krishnan, 1994; Arora, 2001, 2005; Arredondo and Zúñiga, 2004). Differences in the incidence of such diseases between different groups can also throw light on the routes of transmission of the disease (Poundstone, Strathdee, and Celentano, 2004; Pritchett, Thilmany, and Johnson, 2005; Pugliatti, Beghi, Forsgren, Ekman, and Sobocki, 2007). For example, if it is noted that polio is more common in cities in underdeveloped countries, without a clean water supply, than in cities with a good plumbing system, we might advance the theory that polio is spread by the fecal-oral route (Suhrcke, Stuckler, Suk, Desai, Senek, McKee, and Rechel, 2011; Šumilo, Bormane, Asokliene, Vasilenko, Golovljova, Avsic-Zupanc, and Randolph, 2008). Two routes are considered to be airborne: Airborne infections and droplet infections (Bergevoet, Van Schaik, Veling, Backus, and Franken, 2009; Binder, 1988; Bolos, Bacarea, and Marusteri, 2011).

A sexually transmitted infection is any disease that can be caught during sexual activity with another person, including vaginal or anal sex or through oral sex (Arredondo and Zúñiga, 2006; Backer, van Roermund, Fischer, van Asseldonk, and Bergevoet, 2015; Bartsch, Hotez, Hertenstein, Diemert, Zapf, Bottazzi, and Lee, 2016). Transmission can occur directly between surfaces in contact during intercourse (Howe, Häsler, and Stärk, 2013; Howe et al., 2012). This is the usual route for bacterial infections and those infections causing sores (Raut, 2004; Rehm, Mathers, Popova, Thavorncharoensap, Teerawattananon, and Patra, 2009; Rich and Perry, 2011). It can also occur from secretions (semen or the fluid secreted by the excited female) which carry infectious agents that get into the partner's bloodstream through tiny tears in the penis, vagina or rectum (Hart and Halden, 2020; Häsler, Howe, and Stärk, 2011; Henschke, Kamper, and Maher, 2015; Hochberg, 1992). This is a more usual route for viruses (Markos and Abdela, 2016; Martin and Shepherd, 2009; McGuinness, McGlynn, Johnson, MacIntyre, Batty, Burns, and McGinty, 2012). In this second case, anal sex is considerably more hazardous since the penis opens more tears in the rectum than the vagina, as the vagina is more elastic and more accommodating (Foxman, 2002; Garner, Whan, Gard, and Phillips, 2001; Gayle and Hill, 2001; Gottstein, Pozio, and Nöckler, 2009). Some diseases transmissible by the sexual route include HIV/AIDS, chlamydia, genital warts, gonorrhea, hepatitis B, syphilis, herpes, and trichomoniasis (Moné, Ibikounlé, Massougbodji, and Mouahid, 2010; Morand, 2004; Moro, Budke, Schantz, Vasquez, Santivanez, and Villavicencio, 2011).

Sexually transmitted diseases such as HIV and hepatitis B are thought to not normally be transmitted through mouth-to-mouth contact, although it is possible to transmit some STDs between the genitals and the mouth, during oral sex (Eaton and Groopman, 2013; Eckelman, Sherman, and MacNeill, 2018; Egger, 2011; Elbe, 2007; Ernst and Hay, 1994). In the case of HIV, this possibility has been established (Oleś, Gudowska-Nowak, and Kleczkowski, 2012; Otte, Nugent, and McLeod, 2004; Ozawa, Portnoy, Getaneh, Clark,

Knoll, Bishai, and Patwardhan, 2016). It is also responsible for the increased incidence of herpes simplex virus 1 (which is usually responsible for oral infections) in genital infections and the increased incidence of the type 2 virus (more common genitally) in oral infections (Rogers, Carolin, Vaught, and Compton, 2011; Ronohardjo and Rastiko, 1982; Sachs, 2001; Sachs and Malaney, 2002). Diseases that are transmitted primarily by oral means may be caught through direct oral contact such as kissing, or by indirect contact such as by sharing a drinking glass or a cigarette (Bausch and Schwarz, 2014; Bausch et al., 2001; Benner, Carabin, Sánchez-Serrano, Budke, and Carmena, 2010). Diseases that are known to be transmissible by kissing or by other direct or indirect oral contact include all of the diseases transmissible by droplet contact and (at least) all forms of herpes viruses, namely Cytomegalovirus infections, herpes simplex virus (especially HSV-1) and infectious mononucleosis (Purevdawa, Moon, Baigalmaa, Davaajav, Smith, and Vermund, 1997; Ramesh, Malla, Raju, Sehgal, Ganguly, Mahajan, and Dilawari, 1990).

A vector is an organism that does not cause disease itself but that transmits infection by conveying pathogens from one host to another. Vectors may be mechanical or biological (Borghol, Suderman, McArdle, Racine, Hallett, Pembrey, and Szyf, 2012; Brandes, 2008; Brown, Lipscomb, and Snyder, 2001). A mechanical vector picks up an infectious agent on the outside of its body and transmits it in a passive manner (Tapia, 2003; Torgerson and Dowling, 2001; Torgerson, Carmona, and Bonifacino, 2000; Uddin Khan, Atanasova, Krueger, Ramirez, and Gray, 2013). An example of a mechanical vector is a housefly, which lands on cow dung, contaminating its appendages with bacteria from the feces, and then lands on food prior to consumption (Saleha, 1991; Sibert, Rigaud, Delavierre, and Labat, 2010; Skrepnek and Skrepnek, 2004; Sloane, 2009; Sockett, 1993). The pathogen never enters the body of the fly (Peckham, 2013; Perrings et al., 2002, 2014). In contrast, biological vectors harbor pathogens within their bodies and deliver pathogens to new hosts in an active manner, usually a bite (Daily, and Ehrlich, 1996; Deogaonkar, Hutubessy, Van Der Putten, Evers, and Jit, 2012; Dorn, 1992; Ducrotoy, Bertu, Ocholi, Gusi, Bryssinckx, Welburn, and Moriyon, 2014). Biological vectors are often responsible for serious blood-borne diseases, such as malaria, viral encephalitis, Chagas disease, Lyme disease and African sleeping sickness (Fenichel, 2013; Fenichel et al., 2011; Fogel, 1994). Biological vectors are usually, though not exclusively, arthropods, such as mosquitoes, ticks, fleas, and lice (Narrod, Zinsstag, and Tiongco, 2012; Nascimento and de Oliveira, 2014; O'Brien, Lahue,

Caro, and Davidson, 2007). Vectors are often required in the life cycle of a pathogen (Casamassimo, Thikkurissy, Edelstein, and Maiorini, 2009; Castro, Wilson, and Bloom, 2017). A common strategy used to control vector-borne infectious diseases is to interrupt the life cycle of a pathogen by killing the vector (Abegunde and Stanciole, 2008; Abramowitz, Lacau Saint Guily, Moyal-Barracco, Bergeron, Borne, Dahlab, and Bénard, 2018).

In the fecal-oral route, pathogens in fecal particles pass from one person to the mouth of another person (Acemoglu and Johnson, 2007; Adda, 2016; Alloul, Sauriol, Kennedy, Laurier, Tessier, Novosel, and Contandriopoulos, 1998). Although it is usually discussed as a route of transmission, it is actually a specification of the entry and exit portals of the pathogen, and can operate across several of the other routes of transmission (Amuna and Zotor, 2008; Aral, Holmes, Padian, and Cates, 1996; Arbabi, Nezami, Hooshyar, and Delavari, 2018). Fecal-oral transmission is primarily considered as an indirect contact route through contaminated food or water (Armelagos, Brown, and Turner, 2005; Arokiasamy and Krishnan, 1994; Arora, 2001, 2005; Arredondo and Zúñiga, 2004). However, it can also operate through direct contact with feces or contaminated body parts, such as through anal sex (Arredondo and Zúñiga, 2006; Backer, van Roermund, Fischer, van Asseldonk, and Bergevoet, 2015; Bartsch, Hotez, Hertenstein, Diemert, Zapf, Bottazzi, and Lee, 2016). It can also operate through droplet or airborne transmission through the toilet plume from contaminated toilets (Bausch and Schwarz, 2014; Bausch et al., 2001; Benner, Carabin, Sánchez-Serrano, Budke, and Carmena, 2010). Main causes of fecal-oral disease transmission include lack of adequate sanitation and poor hygiene practices, which can take various forms (Bergevoet, Van Schaik, Veling, Backus, and Franken, 2009; Binder, 1988; Bolos, Bacarea, and Marusteri, 2011). Fecal oral transmission can be via foodstuffs or water that has become contaminated (Bonds, Keenan, Rohani, and Sachs, 2010; Boni, Galvani, Wickelgren, and Malani, 2013; Bonovas and Nikolopoulos, 2012). This can happen when people do not adequately wash their hands after using the toilet and before preparing food or tending to patients (Borghol, Suderman, McArdle, Racine, Hallett, Pembrey, and Szyf, 2012; Brandes, 2008; Brown, Lipscomb, and Snyder, 2001).

The fecal-oral route of transmission can be a public health risk for people in developing countries who live in urban slums without access to adequate sanitation (Buckley, 1984; Budke, Jiamin, Qian, and Torgerson, 2005; Bundy, Arámbulo III, and Grey, 1983; Buzby and Roberts, 2009). Here, excreta or untreated sewage can pollute drinking water sources such as groundwater or surface water (Bwire, Munier, Ouedraogo, Heyerdahl, Komakech, Kagirita, and Makumbi, 2017; Canali, Aragrande, Angheben, Capelli, Drigo, Gobbi, and Cassini, 2020). The people who drink the polluted water can become infected (Casamassimo, Thikkurissy, Edelstein, and Maiorini, 2009; Castro, Wilson, and Bloom, 2017). Another problem in some developing countries, is open defecation which leads to disease transmission via the fecal-oral route (Chen, Li, Hsieh, Chang, Lee, Lee, and Ko, 2012; Conover, Pitt, Kessler, DuBow, and Sanborn, 1995; Crump, Murdoch, and Baker, 2001). Even in developed countries there are periodic system failures resulting in a sanitary sewer overflow (Daily, and Ehrlich, 1996; Deogaonkar, Hutubessy, Van Der Putten, Evers, and Jit, 2012; Dorn, 1992; Ducrotoy, Bertu, Ocholi, Gusi, Bryssinckx, Welburn, and Moriyon, 2014). This is the typical mode of transmission for infectious agents such as cholera, hepatitis A, polio, Rotavirus, Salmonella, and parasites such as Ascaris lumbricoides (Eaton and Groopman, 2013; Eckelman, Sherman, and MacNeill, 2018; Egger, 2011; Elbe, 2007; Ernst and Hay, 1994).

Tracking the transmission of infectious diseases is called disease surveillance (Espinoza, Terashima, Herrera-Velit, and Marcos, 2010; Ezzati, Vander Hoorn, Lawes, Leach, James, Lopez, and Murray, 2005). Surveillance of infectious diseases in the public realm traditionally has been the responsibility of public health agencies, either on the national, international or a local level (Fenichel, 2013; Fenichel et al., 2011; Fogel, 1994). Public health staff relies on health care workers and microbiology laboratories to report cases of reportable diseases to them (Foxman, 2002; Garner, Whan, Gard, and Phillips, 2001; Gayle and Hill, 2001; Gottstein, Pozio, and Nöckler, 2009). The analysis of aggregate data can show the spread of a disease and is at the core of the specialty of epidemiology (Hart and Halden, 2020; Häsler, Howe, and Stärk, 2011; Henschke, Kamper, and Maher, 2015; Hochberg, 1992). To understand the spread of the vast majority of non-notifiable diseases, data either need to be collected in a particular study, or existing data collections can be mined, such as insurance company data or antimicrobial drug sales for example (Howe, Häsler, and Stärk, 2013; Howe et al., 2012). For diseases transmitted within an institution (such as a hospital, prison, nursing home, boarding school, orphanage, refugee camp, etc.), infection control specialists are employed, who will review medical records to analyze transmission as part of a hospital epidemiology program, for example (Jenkins, Baingana, Ahmad, McDaid, and Atun, 2011; Johnson, Alvarez-Pasquin, Bijl, Franco, Gaillat, Clara, and Weinke, 2015).

Because these traditional methods are slow, time-consuming, and labor-intensive, proxies of transmission have been sought (Kim and Goldie, 2008; Klein, Laxminarayan, Smith, and Gilligan, 2007; Klepac, Laxminarayan, and Grenfell, 2011). One proxy in the case of influenza is tracking of influenza-like illness at certain sentinel sites of health care practitioners within a state, for example (Krieger, 2001a, b; Lemma, 1969; Liu, Maniadakis, Gray, and Rayner, 2002; López, Torné, Franco, San-Martin, Viayna, Barrull, and Perulero, 2018). Tools have been developed to help track influenza epidemics by finding patterns in certain web search query activity (Markos and Abdela, 2016; Martin and Shepherd, 2009; McGuinness, McGlynn, Johnson, MacIntyre, Batty, Burns, and McGinty, 2012). It was found that the frequency of influenza-related web searches as a whole; rises as the number of people sick with influenza rises (Moné, Ibikounlé, Massougbodji, and Mouahid, 2010; Morand, 2004; Moro, Budke, Schantz, Vasquez, Santivanez, and Villavicencio, 2011). Examining space-time relationships of web queries has been shown to approximate the spread of influenza and dengue (Narrod, Zinsstag, and Tiongco, 2012; Nascimento and de Oliveira, 2014; O'Brien, Lahue, Caro, and Davidson, 2007). Computer simulations of infectious disease spread have been used (Oleś, Gudowska-Nowak, and Kleczkowski, 2012; Otte, Nugent, and McLeod, 2004; Ozawa, Portnoy, Getaneh, Clark, Knoll, Bishai, and Patwardhan, 2016). Human aggregation can drive transmission, seasonal variation and outbreaks of infectious diseases, such as the annual start of school, boot camp, the annual Hajj, and similar events (Ozmen, Kurşun, and Ozcelik, 2005; Paarlberg, Hillberg, Lee, and Mathews, 2008; Paisley, Vraa-Andersen, Dybkjaer, Møller, Christensen, Mousing, and Agger, 1993). Most recently, data from cell phones have been shown to be able to capture population movements well enough to predict the transmission of certain infectious diseases, like rubella (Pal, Kerorsa, Marami, and Kandi, 2020; Paterson, Otte, Slingenbergh, Wint, and Rogers, 2000; Pearce and Merletti, 2006).

Pathogens must have a way to be transmitted from one host to another to ensure their species' survival (Peckham, 2013; Perrings et al., 2002, 2014). Infectious agents are generally specialized for a particular method of transmission (Perry and Randolph, 1999; Philipson, 2000; Philipson and Posner, 1996; Pongchaiyakul, Songpattanasilp, and Taechakraichana, 2008). Taking an example from the respiratory route, from an evolutionary perspective viruses or bacteria that cause their host to develop coughing and sneezing symptoms have a great survival advantage, as they are much more likely to be ejected from one host and carried to another (Poundstone,

Strathdee, and Celentano, 2004; Pritchett, Thilmany, and Johnson, 2005; Pugliatti, Beghi, Forsgren, Ekman, and Sobocki, 2007). This is also the reason that many microorganisms cause diarrhea (Purevdawa, Moon, Baigalmaa, Davaajav, Smith, and Vermund, 1997; Ramesh, Malla, Raju, Sehgal, Ganguly, Mahajan, and Dilawari, 1990). The relationship between virulence and transmission is complex and has important consequences for the long-term evolution of a pathogen (Raut, 2004; Rehm, Mathers, Popova, Thavorncharoensap, Teerawattananon, and Patra, 2009; Rich and Perry, 2011). Since it takes many generations for a microbe and a new host species to co-evolve, an emerging pathogen may hit its earliest victims especially hard (Rogers, Carolin, Vaught, and Compton, 2011; Ronohardjo and Rastiko, 1982; Sachs, 2001; Sachs and Malaney, 2002). It is usually in the first wave of a new disease that death rates are highest (Saleha, 1991; Sibert, Rigaud, Delavierre, and Labat, 2010; Skrepnek and Skrepnek, 2004; Sloane, 2009; Sockett, 1993). If a disease is rapidly fatal, the host may die before the microbe can be passed along to another host (St George, 1986; Steben and Duarte-Franco, 2007; Stehr-Green and Schantz, 1987; Stuckler, 2008; Stuckler and Siegel, 2011). However, this cost may be overwhelmed by the short-term benefit of higher infectiousness if transmission is linked to virulence, as it is for instance in the case of cholera (the explosive diarrhea aids the bacterium in finding new hosts) or many respiratory infections such as sneezing and coughing create infectious aerosols (Suhrcke, Stuckler, Suk, Desai, Senek, McKee, and Rechel, 2011; Šumilo, Bormane, Asokliene, Vasilenko, Golovljova, Avsic-Zupanc, and Randolph, 2008). The next section considers the classification of epidemics by the era in which they occur.

4.4. CLASSIFICATION OF DISEASE EPIDEMICS BY ERA IN WHICH THEY OCCUR

One of the ways in which disease epidemicsDisease epidemics can be classified is through reference to the era within which they occurred (Uusküla, Müürsepp, Kawai, Raag, Jürisson, and Pillsbury, 2013; Vanni, Karnon, Madan, White, Edmunds, Foss, and Legood, 2011). However, this is not always an exact science since many epidemics sporadically appear and reappear. For the most part, this type of classification is for historical purposes (Weycker, Edelsberg, Oster, and Tino, 2005; Wu, Perrings, Kinzig, Collins, Minteer, and Daszak, 2017; Yach, Stuckler, and Brownell, 2006). For example, in this section we can focus on those epidemics and the major events surrounding them (Yi-Xin and Manderson, 2005; Zadoks, 2008; Zhan, Li, Wang, Sun, Geng, Xiong, and de Hoog, 2015; Zhang, Song, Cai, and Zhou, 2008). This roughly translates in the period from 1900 and 2000 with a few decades on either end (Casamassimo, Thikkurissy, Edelstein, and Maiorini, 2009; Castro, Wilson, and Bloom, 2017). The latest is the COVID-19 crisis which has had significant impacts on the economy. Figure 4.4 is an example of a conceptual model that can be used to predict disease epidemicsDisease epidemics based on the characteristics of a population and past experiences.

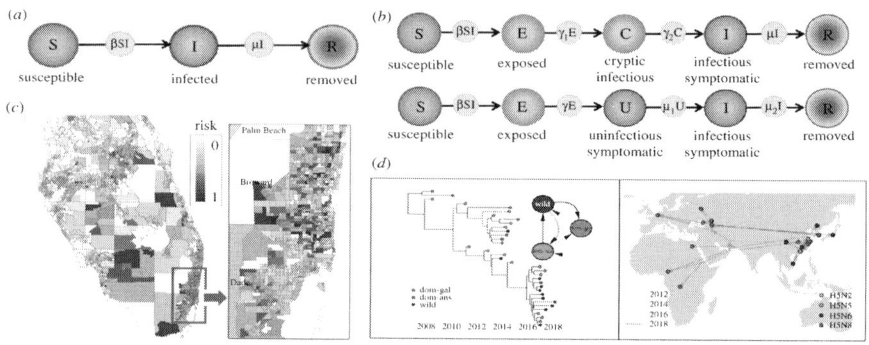

Figure 4.4. Conceptual model for forecasting disease epidemics.

Source: Royal Society Publishing.

Here is a summary of some of the key events relating to global epidemiology from 1899 to 2020:

- **1899 to 1923:** A new outbreak of cholera, a bacterial infection contracted through the consumption of contaminated food and water, begins in India at the turn of the century (Narrod, Zinsstag, and Tiongco, 2012; Nascimento and de Oliveira, 2014; O'Brien, Lahue, Caro, and Davidson, 2007). It is the latest wave of a disease that has caused pandemics intermittently since the early 1800s (Fenichel, 2013; Fenichel et al., 2011; Fogel, 1994). The outbreak spreads to Russia, as well as to parts of the Middle East and North Africa, ultimately killing hundreds of thousands of people (Daily, and Ehrlich, 1996; Deogaonkar, Hutubessy, Van Der Putten, Evers, and Jit, 2012; Dorn, 1992; Ducrotoy, Bertu, Ocholi, Gusi, Bryssinckx, Welburn, and Moriyon, 2014). There are particularly high death tolls in India and Russia (Peckham, 2013; Perrings et al., 2002, 2014). Advancements in sanitation and public hygiene are credited with preventing the pandemic from taking hold in Europe and North America (Saleha, 1991; Sibert, Rigaud, Delavierre, and Labat, 2010; Skrepnek and Skrepnek, 2004; Sloane, 2009; Sockett, 1993).

- **1918 to 1920:** A new influenza virus begins to spread worldwide amid the upheavals of World War I (Tapia, 2003; Torgerson and Dowling, 2001; Torgerson, Carmona, and Bonifacino, 2000; Uddin Khan, Atanasova, Krueger, Ramirez, and Gray, 2013). There is no consensus on the origin of the pandemic, but it is first publicly reported in Spain (Borghol, Suderman, McArdle, Racine, Hallett, Pembrey, and Szyf, 2012; Brandes, 2008; Brown, Lipscomb, and Snyder, 2001). It infects an estimated 500 million people, roughly one-third of the world's population at the time, and kills some 50 million, with an unusually high fatality rate among otherwise healthy young adults (Purevdawa, Moon, Baigalmaa, Davaajav, Smith, and Vermund, 1997; Ramesh, Malla, Raju, Sehgal, Ganguly, Mahajan, and Dilawari, 1990). Many governments look to isolation measures, quarantines, and disinfecting efforts, but the global movement of troops hinders containment (Bausch and Schwarz, 2014; Bausch et al., 2001; Benner, Carabin, Sánchez-Serrano, Budke, and Carmena, 2010). At the time, there is no flu vaccine and antibiotics have not yet been developed to treat secondary bacterial infections (Rogers, Carolin, Vaught, and Compton, 2011; Ronohardjo and Rastiko, 1982; Sachs, 2001; Sachs and Malaney, 2002). In the United States alone, about 675,000 people die, lowering the country's average life expectancy by more than 12 years (Oleś, Gudowska-Nowak, and Kleczkowski, 2012; Otte, Nugent, and McLeod, 2004; Ozawa, Portnoy, Getaneh, Clark, Knoll, Bishai, and Patwardhan, 2016).
- **1928 to 1930 and Beyond:** Scottish scientist Alexander Fleming discovers penicillin, the first antibiotic, a class of drugs used to treat bacterial infection (Eaton and Groopman, 2013; Eckelman, Sherman, and MacNeill, 2018; Egger, 2011; Elbe, 2007; Ernst and Hay, 1994). Hence, this marked a major milestone for global health (Moné, Ibikounlé, Massougbodji, and Mouahid, 2010; Morand, 2004; Moro, Budke, Schantz, Vasquez, Santivanez, and Villavicencio, 2011). Widespread use of antibiotics takes off in the early 1940s during World War II (Foxman, 2002; Garner, Whan,

Gard, and Phillips, 2001; Gayle and Hill, 2001; Gottstein, Pozio, and Nöckler, 2009). They soon become the go-to treatment for common illnesses, such as strep throat and urinary tract infections, and significantly reduce the death rates for many ailments, including syphilis and tuberculosis (Markos and Abdela, 2016; Martin and Shepherd, 2009; McGuinness, McGlynn, Johnson, MacIntyre, Batty, Burns, and McGinty, 2012).

- **1948 and Beyond:** The WHO's constitution, signed by more than 60 countries, enters into force in April 1948 (Hart and Halden, 2020; Häsler, Howe, and Stärk, 2011; Henschke, Kamper, and Maher, 2015; Hochberg, 1992). The body, a part of the newly formed United Nations, sets out to coordinate international health policy, seeking to combat diseases such as malaria and tuberculosis and improve sanitation practices (Raut, 2004; Rehm, Mathers, Popova, Thavorncharoensap, Teerawattananon, and Patra, 2009; Rich and Perry, 2011). The WHO builds on previous agencies including the League of Nations' Health Organization (1920–1948), as well as earlier initiatives such as the International Sanitary Conferences, the Pan American Health Organization, and the International Office of Public Hygiene; which beginning in the 19th century issued regulations to improve health standards and prevent the spread of diseases such as cholera and yellow fever (Howe, Häsler, and Stärk, 2013; Howe et al., 2012).
- **1957 to 1958:** A new strain of influenza virus, designated H2N2, is reported in Singapore in February 1957, and soon spreads to China, Hong Kong, the United Kingdom, and the United States (Arredondo and Zúñiga, 2006; Backer, van Roermund, Fischer, van Asseldonk, and Bergevoet, 2015; Bartsch, Hotez, Hertenstein, Diemert, Zapf, Bottazzi, and Lee, 2016). Though less severe than the Spanish Flu, the Asian Flu kills more than 1 million people worldwide (Bergevoet, Van Schaik, Veling, Backus, and Franken, 2009; Binder, 1988; Bolos, Bacarea, and Marusteri, 2011). A second wave of cases beginning at the end of that year is particularly deadly, and young children, elderly people, and pregnant women are hardest hit (Suhrcke, Stuckler, Suk, Desai, Senek, McKee, and Rechel, 2011; Šumilo, Bormane, Asokliene, Vasilenko, Golovljova, Avsic-Zupanc, and Randolph, 2008). A vaccine is quickly developed in 1957, but its deployment is limited and it does little to mitigate the outbreak, experts later

say (Poundstone, Strathdee, and Celentano, 2004; Pritchett, Thilmany, and Johnson, 2005; Pugliatti, Beghi, Forsgren, Ekman, and Sobocki, 2007).

- **1961 and Beyond:** A cholera pandemic originating in Indonesia spreads to other parts of Asia, the Middle East, and Africa over the course of a decade, and continues to this day (Armelagos, Brown, and Turner, 2005; Arokiasamy and Krishnan, 1994; Arora, 2001, 2005; Arredondo and Zúñiga, 2004). By the 1990s outbreaks also take hold in South America, the first on that continent in nearly a century (Krieger, 2001a, b; Lemma, 1969; Liu, Maniadakis, Gray, and Rayner, 2002; López, Torné, Franco, San-Martin, Viayna, Barrull, and Perulero, 2018). An outbreak in Zimbabwe in 2008–09 kills more than 4000 people, and major outbreaks in Haiti and Yemen each affect more than a half-million people (Amuna and Zotor, 2008; Aral, Holmes, Padian, and Cates, 1996; Arbabi, Nezami, Hooshyar, and Delavari, 2018). Some 3 million people are infected with the bacteria that cause cholera each year, and it remains endemic in close to 50 countries (Acemoglu and Johnson, 2007; Adda, 2016; Alloul, Sauriol, Kennedy, Laurier, Tessier, Novosel, and Contandriopoulos, 1998). Health experts say oral cholera vaccines, introduced in the 1990s, are not a replacement for improved sanitation (St George, 1986; Steben and Duarte-Franco, 2007; Stehr-Green and Schantz, 1987; Stuckler, 2008; Stuckler and Siegel, 2011).
- **1968 to 1969:** A decade after the Asian Flu, a new strain called H3N2 emerges. Commonly called the Hong Kong Flu, it emerges first in Hong Kong, then a British colony, in July 1968 (Uusküla, Müürsepp, Kawai, Raag, Jürisson, and Pillsbury, 2013; Vanni, Karnon, Madan, White, Edmunds, Foss, and Legood, 2011). It soon travels across East and South Asia, then to Australia, Europe, and North America, and on to Africa and South America by 1969 (Perry and Randolph, 1999; Philipson, 2000; Philipson and Posner, 1996; Pongchaiyakul, Songpattanasilp, and Taechakraichana, 2008). U.S. troops returning from the Vietnam War are believed to have brought the virus to the United States (Weycker, Edelsberg, Oster, and Tino, 2005; Wu, Perrings, Kinzig, Collins, Minteer, and Daszak, 2017; Yach, Stuckler, and Brownell, 2006). An estimated 1 million people die in the pandemic, about half of them from Hong Kong and many of them

people 65 years of age or older (Chen, Li, Hsieh, Chang, Lee, Lee, and Ko, 2012; Conover, Pitt, Kessler, DuBow, and Sanborn, 1995; Crump, Murdoch, and Baker, 2001). Descendants of the H3N2 virus continue to circulate seasonally worldwide (Kim and Goldie, 2008; Klein, Laxminarayan, Smith, and Gilligan, 2007; Klepac, Laxminarayan, and Grenfell, 2011).

- **1977 to 1980:** The last known case of smallpox, a viral disease that plagued humans for millennia, is diagnosed in 1977 in Somalia, following a nearly two-decade-long global vaccination campaign (Abegunde and Stanciole, 2008; Abramowitz, Lacau Saint Guily, Moyal-Barracco, Bergeron, Borne, Dahlab, and Bénard, 2018). Three years later the WHO formally declares it eradicated around the globe (Jenkins, Baingana, Ahmad, McDaid, and Atun, 2011; Johnson, Alvarez-Pasquin, Bijl, Franco, Gaillat, Clara, and Weinke, 2015). The elimination of the disease, which was fatal in as many as one-third of patients, marks unusual U.S.-Soviet cooperation during the Cold War (Pal, Kerorsa, Marami, and Kandi, 2020; Paterson, Otte, Slingenbergh, Wint, and Rogers, 2000; Pearce and Merletti, 2006). It also highlights major advancements in the study and use of vaccines: polio vaccines introduced in the 1950s and 1960s lead to similar success globally (Yi-Xin and Manderson, 2005; Zadoks, 2008; Zhan, Li, Wang, Sun, Geng, Xiong, and de Hoog, 2015; Zhang, Song, Cai, and Zhou, 2008). Vaccines are credited with reducing rates of illnesses such as measles, diphtheria, and whooping cough to all-time lows (Bwire, Munier, Ouedraogo, Heyerdahl, Komakech, Kagirita, and Makumbi, 2017; Canali, Aragrande, Angheben, Capelli, Drigo, Gobbi, and Cassini, 2020).
- **1981 and Beyond:** A 1981 report by what is now the U.S. Centers for Disease Control and Prevention (CDC) describes a rare form of pneumonia that is later identified as Acquired Immunodeficiency Syndrome, or AIDS (Buckley, 1984; Budke, Jiamin, Qian, and Torgerson, 2005; Bundy, Arámbulo III, and Grey, 1983; Buzby and Roberts, 2009). It is the most advanced stage of human immunodeficiency virus (HIV). This marks the start of an explosive growth of cases, and by the early 1990s AIDS becomes the leading cause of death in men between the ages of 25 and 44 in the United States (Espinoza, Terashima, Herrera-Velit, and Marcos, 2010; Ezzati, Vander Hoorn, Lawes,

Leach, James, Lopez, and Murray, 2005). In 1996, the United Nations establishes UNAIDS to coordinate global action (Bonds, Keenan, Rohani, and Sachs, 2010; Boni, Galvani, Wickelgren, and Malani, 2013; Bonovas and Nikolopoulos, 2012). The introduction of antiretroviral therapy helps to bring down the U.S. death toll, but the epidemic grows across Africa (Ozmen, Kurşun, and Ozcelik, 2005; Paarlberg, Hillberg, Lee, and Mathews, 2008; Paisley, Vraa-Andersen, Dybkjaer, Møller, Christensen, Mousing, and Agger, 1993). The 2003; U.S. president's emergency plan for AIDS Relief (PEPFAR) boosts international funding, and between 2000 and 2018; HIV-related deaths decrease by 45% (Casamassimo, Thikkurissy, Edelstein, and Maiorini, 2009; Castro, Wilson, and Bloom, 2017). Today, close to 40 million people have HIV/AIDS, more than two-thirds of whom are in sub-Saharan Africa (Poundstone, Strathdee, and Celentano, 2004; Pritchett, Thilmany, and Johnson, 2005; Pugliatti, Beghi, Forsgren, Ekman, and Sobocki, 2007). Tens of millions of people have died from the disease.

- **2002 to 2003:** The severe acute respiratory syndrome (SARS) coronavirus, part of a family of viruses that commonly cause respiratory symptoms such as coughing and shortness of breath, is first identified in late 2002 in southern China (St George, 1986; Steben and Duarte-Franco, 2007; Stehr-Green and Schantz, 1987; Stuckler, 2008; Stuckler and Siegel, 2011). SARS spreads to more than two dozen countries across four continents, infecting more than 8000 people (Kim and Goldie, 2008; Klein, Laxminarayan, Smith, and Gilligan, 2007; Klepac, Laxminarayan, and Grenfell, 2011). In March 2003, the WHO triggers its global outbreak alert and response network (GOARN) to coordinate research by teams of international experts and the deployment of supplies and health workers to affected countries (Bonds, Keenan, Rohani, and Sachs, 2010; Boni, Galvani, Wickelgren, and Malani, 2013; Bonovas and Nikolopoulos, 2012). Health experts sharply criticize Beijing for covering up the initial spread of the virus. SARS kills close to 800, most within China and Hong Kong, by the time the outbreak is quelled in mid-2003 (Oleś, Gudowska-Nowak, and Kleczkowski, 2012; Otte, Nugent, and McLeod, 2004; Ozawa, Portnoy, Getaneh, Clark, Knoll, Bishai, and Patwardhan, 2016). The virus is thought to have been transmitted to humans via contact with civet cats (Armelagos, Brown, and Turner, 2005; Arokiasamy and Krishnan, 1994; Arora, 2001, 2005; Arredondo and Zúñiga, 2004).

- **2005 and Beyond:** The WHO rewrites its International Health Regulations, rules originally drawn up in 1969 that are binding on all WHO member states (Bwire, Munier, Ouedraogo, Heyerdahl, Komakech, Kagirita, and Makumbi, 2017; Canali, Aragrande, Angheben, Capelli, Drigo, Gobbi, and Cassini, 2020). The new rules aim to boost collective defenses against global health challenges and improve pandemic preparedness and response (Borghol, Suderman, McArdle, Racine, Hallett, Pembrey, and Szyf, 2012; Brandes, 2008; Brown, Lipscomb, and Snyder, 2001). Entering into force in June 2007, they require states to notify the WHO of potential global health emergencies (Peckham, 2013; Perrings et al., 2002, 2014). They also grant the WHO director-general the authority to declare a public health emergency of international concern, or PHEIC, in order to mobilize a global response (Amuna and Zotor, 2008; Aral, Holmes, Padian, and Cates, 1996; Arbabi, Nezami, Hooshyar, and Delavari, 2018). The changes are meant to build on the GOARN established in 2000 (Acemoglu and Johnson, 2007; Adda, 2016; Alloul, Sauriol, Kennedy, Laurier, Tessier, Novosel, and Contandriopoulos, 1998).
- **2009 to 2010:** A new influenza virus, labeled H1N1 and commonly referred to as the swine flu because of its links to influenza viruses that circulate in pigs, begins to spread in early 2009 in Mexico and the United States (Eaton and Groopman, 2013; Eckelman, Sherman, and MacNeill, 2018; Egger, 2011; Elbe, 2007; Ernst and Hay, 1994). Unlike other strains of influenza, H1N1 disproportionately affects children and younger people (Espinoza, Terashima, Herrera-Velit, and Marcos, 2010; Ezzati, Vander Hoorn, Lawes, Leach, James, Lopez, and Murray, 2005). The CDC calls it the first global flu pandemic in 40 years (Markos and Abdela, 2016; Martin and Shepherd, 2009; McGuinness, McGlynn, Johnson, MacIntyre, Batty, Burns, and McGinty, 2012). The WHO declares a PHEIC in April 2009, then designates the spread of H1N1 a pandemic in June, after the virus reaches more than 70 countries (Suhrcke, Stuckler, Suk, Desai, Senek, McKee, and Rechel, 2011; Šumilo, Bormane,

Asokliene, Vasilenko, Golovljova, Avsic-Zupanc, and Randolph, 2008). In response, some countries advise against travel to North America, and China imposes mandatory quarantines for patients and their close contacts (Bergevoet, Van Schaik, Veling, Backus, and Franken, 2009; Binder, 1988; Bolos, Bacarea, and Marusteri, 2011). The CDC estimates that between 151,700 and 575,400 people die worldwide, around 12,500 in the United States, in the first year after the virus is discovered (Tapia, 2003; Torgerson and Dowling, 2001; Torgerson, Carmona, and Bonifacino, 2000; Uddin Khan, Atanasova, Krueger, Ramirez, and Gray, 2013). Around 80% of those who die are younger than 65 (Moné, Ibikounlé, Massougbodji, and Mouahid, 2010; Morand, 2004; Moro, Budke, Schantz, Vasquez, Santivanez, and Villavicencio, 2011). The WHO announces the pandemic's end in August 2010, though the strain continues to circulate seasonally (Uusküla, Müürsepp, Kawai, Raag, Jürisson, and Pillsbury, 2013; Vanni, Karnon, Madan, White, Edmunds, Foss, and Legood, 2011).

- **2012 and Beyond:** A new coronavirus, named middle east respiratory syndrome (MERS), is transmitted to humans from camels in 2012 in Saudi Arabia (Raut, 2004; Rehm, Mathers, Popova, Thavorncharoensap, Teerawattananon, and Patra, 2009; Rich and Perry, 2011). The largest outbreak occurs on the Arabian Peninsula in the first half of 2014, with the Saudi city of Jeddah as its epicenter (Foxman, 2002; Garner, Whan, Gard, and Phillips, 2001; Gayle and Hill, 2001; Gottstein, Pozio, and Nöckler, 2009). In 2015, South Korea is home to the second-largest outbreak (Howe, Häsler, and Stärk, 2013; Howe et al., 2012). More than two dozen countries report cases of the viral respiratory disease in the following years, though the majority of cases are in Saudi Arabia (Weycker, Edelsberg, Oster, and Tino, 2005; Wu, Perrings, Kinzig, Collins, Minteer, and Daszak, 2017; Yach, Stuckler, and Brownell, 2006). The virus commonly causes pneumonia in those infected and has a relatively high fatality rate: of the roughly 2,500 people diagnosed with MERS since its discovery, more than 850 have died from the disease (Daily, and Ehrlich, 1996; Deogaonkar, Hutubessy, Van Der Putten, Evers, and Jit, 2012; Dorn, 1992; Ducrotoy, Bertu, Ocholi, Gusi, Bryssinckx, Welburn, and Moriyon, 2014).

- **2014 and Beyond:** In May 2014, WHO Director-General Margaret Chan declares a PHEIC over a rise in polio cases in Africa and Asia (Chen, Li, Hsieh, Chang, Lee, Lee, and Ko, 2012; Conover, Pitt, Kessler, DuBow, and Sanborn, 1995; Crump, Murdoch, and Baker, 2001). The virus, which paralyzed or killed a half million people yearly at its peak in the early 1950s, had been nearly eradicated after mass vaccination campaigns starting in the late 1950s (Arredondo and Zúñiga, 2006; Backer, van Roermund, Fischer, van Asseldonk, and Bergevoet, 2015; Bartsch, Hotez, Hertenstein, Diemert, Zapf, Bottazzi, and Lee, 2016). The disease, which disproportionately affects young people, proves hard to eliminate completely, particularly in conflict zones (Rogers, Carolin, Vaught, and Compton, 2011; Ronohardjo and Rastiko, 1982; Sachs, 2001; Sachs and Malaney, 2002). Widespread mistrust of vaccination programs is a major challenge (Yi-Xin and Manderson, 2005; Zadoks, 2008; Zhan, Li, Wang, Sun, Geng, Xiong, and de Hoog, 2015; Zhang, Song, Cai, and Zhou, 2008). As of early 2020, the PHEIC over the possible spread of polio remains in place, and the disease is still endemic in three countries: Afghanistan, Nigeria, and Pakistan (Perry and Randolph, 1999; Philipson, 2000; Philipson and Posner, 1996; Pongchaiyakul, Songpattanasilp, and Taechakraichana, 2008).
- **2014 to 2016:** In early 2014, cases of the Ebola virus, a rare and severe infectious disease that leads to death in roughly half of those who contract it, are detected in Guinea and soon after in Liberia and Sierra Leone (Abegunde and Stanciole, 2008; Abramowitz, Lacau Saint Guily, Moyal-Barracco, Bergeron, Borne, Dahlab, and Bénard, 2018). It is the first time the disease moves into densely populated urban areas, allowing for rapid transmission (Fenichel, 2013; Fenichel et al., 2011; Fogel, 1994). The outbreak eventually spreads to seven other countries, including several European states and the United States, causing more than 11000 deaths in all (Saleha, 1991; Sibert, Rigaud, Delavierre, and Labat, 2010; Skrepnek and Skrepnek, 2004; Sloane, 2009; Sockett, 1993). Mistrust of health workers and rumors again present challenges to containment (Bausch and Schwarz, 2014; Bausch et al., 2001; Benner, Carabin, Sánchez-Serrano, Budke, and Carmena, 2010). The WHO, which declares the outbreak a PHEIC in August 2014, is criticized for what many call a slow

response (Hart and Halden, 2020; Häsler, Howe, and Stärk, 2011; Henschke, Kamper, and Maher, 2015; Hochberg, 1992). In September 2014, the UN Security Council adopted a resolution calling on member states to pool global resources to combat the crisis, and countries including the United States and the United Kingdom, deploy health workers and other aid (Ozmen, Kurşun, and Ozcelik, 2005; Paarlberg, Hillberg, Lee, and Mathews, 2008; Paisley, Vraa-Andersen, Dybkjaer, Møller, Christensen, Mousing, and Agger, 1993). The hardest-hit countries declared themselves Ebola-free in June 2016.

- **2015 and Beyond:** The WHO reports in 2015 that malaria infections are down by more than one-third globally compared to 2000, as the United Nations and the Bill and Melinda Gates Foundation, launched a major joint effort to eradicate the disease by 2040 (Buckley, 1984; Budke, Jiamin, Qian, and Torgerson, 2005; Bundy, Arámbulo III, and Grey, 1983; Buzby and Roberts, 2009). Malaria still kills several hundred thousand people yearly, two-thirds of whom are children under five (Pal, Kerorsa, Marami, and Kandi, 2020; Paterson, Otte, Slingenbergh, Wint, and Rogers, 2000; Pearce and Merletti, 2006). Eradication efforts focus on the 11 countries where the large majority of malaria cases occur, all of which are in sub-Saharan Africa except for India (Narrod, Zinsstag, and Tiongco, 2012; Nascimento and de Oliveira, 2014; O'Brien, Lahue, Caro, and Davidson, 2007). Meanwhile, cases of dengue, another mosquito-borne disease, spike between 2000 and 2015, partly due to increased reporting (Krieger, 2001a, b; Lemma, 1969; Liu, Maniadakis, Gray, and Rayner, 2002; López, Torné, Franco, San-Martin, Viayna, Barrull, and Perulero, 2018). Dengue is endemic in more than 100 countries, with the majority of the 100–400 million yearly cases occurring in Asia (Jenkins, Baingana, Ahmad, McDaid, and Atun, 2011; Johnson, Alvarez-Pasquin, Bijl, Franco, Gaillat, Clara, and Weinke, 2015). These diseases have proven difficult to eliminate, as researchers confront numerous challenges to developing successful vaccines (Purevdawa, Moon, Baigalmaa, Davaajav, Smith, and Vermund, 1997; Ramesh, Malla, Raju, Sehgal, Ganguly, Mahajan, and Dilawari, 1990).
- **2015 to 2016:** An outbreak of the Zika virus, first discovered in Uganda in the 1940s and transmitted mainly by mosquitoes, takes

off in Brazil in early 2015 (Jenkins, Baingana, Ahmad, McDaid, and Atun, 2011; Johnson, Alvarez-Pasquin, Bijl, Franco, Gaillat, Clara, and Weinke, 2015). In February 2016, the WHO declares the outbreak a PHEIC, and by the middle of the year more than 60 countries report cases of the virus, including the United States (Krieger, 2001a, b; Lemma, 1969; Liu, Maniadakis, Gray, and Rayner, 2002; López, Torné, Franco, San-Martin, Viayna, Barrull, and Perulero, 2018). Thousands of women infected with the virus while pregnant give birth to babies with microcephaly, a condition in which a child's head is smaller than normal, and other congenital conditions (Narrod, Zinsstag, and Tiongco, 2012; Nascimento and de Oliveira, 2014; O'Brien, Lahue, Caro, and Davidson, 2007). Some governments urge women to delay pregnancy amid the outbreak (Pal, Kerorsa, Marami, and Kandi, 2020; Paterson, Otte, Slingenbergh, Wint, and Rogers, 2000; Pearce and Merletti, 2006). Despite calls for cancellation, 2016; Summer Olympics in Rio de Janeiro go ahead as planned (Buckley, 1984; Budke, Jiamin, Qian, and Torgerson, 2005; Bundy, Arámbulo III, and Grey, 1983; Buzby and Roberts, 2009). The WHO declared the end of the epidemic in November 2016.

- **2018 and Beyond:** In August 2018, the Democratic Republic of Congo declares an outbreak of the Ebola virus in the country's northeast. Several cases are later reported across the border in Uganda. Protracted conflict in the area hampers the response, as health workers face attacks by armed groups; misinformation and mistrust among the local population are also challenges. By June 2019, the Ebola outbreak becomes the second largest in history, and in July, the WHO declares a PHEIC, urging increased international support to end the crisis. More than 3,400 people are infected with the virus, and more than 2,200 died. By early 2020, the outbreak appears to be winding down, with no new cases reported after mid-February.
- **2019 and Beyond:** A new coronavirus emerges in China's Hubei Province in late 2019, spreading rapidly to other parts of China and infecting tens of thousands of people. The disease soon travels to other parts of Asia and the rest of the world, and in late January 2020, the WHO declares a PHEIC. By March, the virus reaches more than 100 countries, leading the WHO to designate the outbreak a pandemic. Many governments impose

travel restrictions, quarantines, and lockdowns to try to stop its spread. Iran and Italy become hotspots, with these countries reporting among the highest death tolls outside China. More than 10 million cases had been identified by the middle of the year, with about 20% case fatalities.

This chapter will close by looking at the classification of disease epidemicsDisease epidemics based on their level of severity.

4.5. CLASSIFICATION OF DISEASE EPIDEMICS BY THEIR SEVERITY

The severity of illness (SOI) is defined as the extent of organ system derangement or physiologic decompensation for a patient (Ozmen, Kurşun, and Ozcelik, 2005; Paarlberg, Hillberg, Lee, and Mathews, 2008; Paisley, Vraa-Andersen, Dybkjaer, Møller, Christensen, Mousing, and Agger, 1993). It gives a medical classification into minor, moderate, major, and extreme (Hart and Halden, 2020; Häsler, Howe, and Stärk, 2011; Henschke, Kamper, and Maher, 2015; Hochberg, 1992). The SOI class is meant to provide a basis for evaluating hospital resource use or to establish patient care guidelines (Bausch and Schwarz, 2014; Bausch et al., 2001; Benner, Carabin, Sánchez-Serrano, Budke, and Carmena, 2010). Patients are assigned their SOI based on their specific diagnoses and procedures performed during their medical encounter, which is generally an inpatient hospital stay (Saleha, 1991; Sibert, Rigaud, Delavierre, and Labat, 2010; Skrepnek and Skrepnek, 2004; Sloane, 2009; Sockett, 1993). Patients with higher SOI (e.g., major or extreme) are more likely to consume greater healthcare resources and stay longer in hospitals than patients with lower SOI in the same diagnosis-related group or DRG (Fenichel, 2013; Fenichel et al., 2011; Fogel, 1994). However, it is also important to note that any epidemic (regardless of its severity) can have far-reaching effects because of its interaction implications (see Figure 4.5).

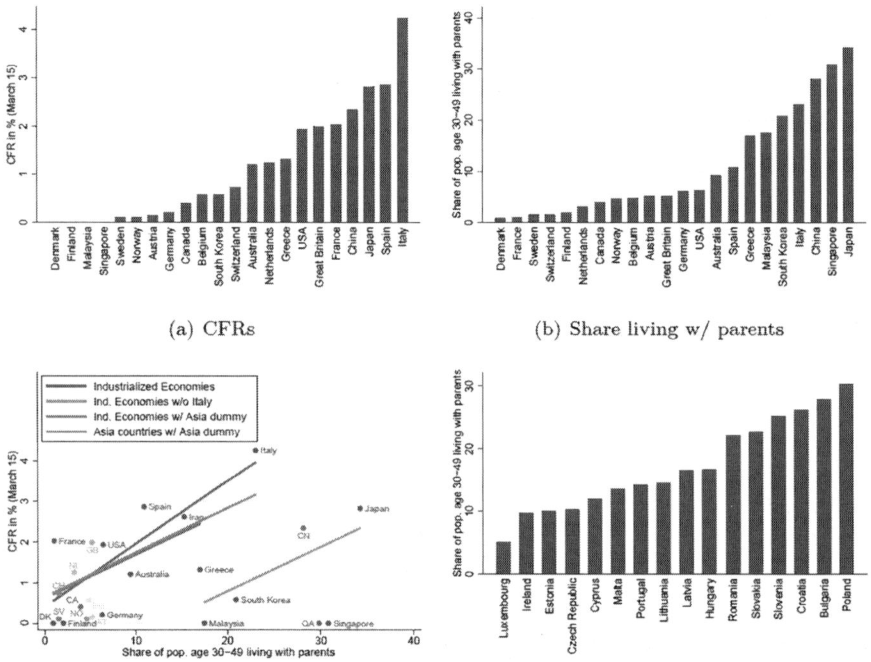

(a) CFRs

(b) Share living w/ parents

(c) Vertical social interaction and CFRs

(d) Share living w/ parents further EU countries

Figure 4.5. Important social interaction frameworks during epidemics.

Source: Centre for Economic Policy Research.

The Centers for Medicare and Medicaid Services considered the 3M APR-DRG and SOI system as a potential evolution to the DRG system in 2006 (Yi-Xin and Manderson, 2005; Zadoks, 2008; Zhan, Li, Wang, Sun, Geng, Xiong, and de Hoog, 2015; Zhang, Song, Cai, and Zhou, 2008). However, it received such negative feedback from the industry that in March 2007 decided to adopt another internally developed system evolved from the DRG (Perry and Randolph, 1999; Philipson, 2000; Philipson and Posner, 1996; Pongchaiyakul, Songpattanasilp, and Taechakraichana, 2008). SOI is still commonly used throughout the United States to adjust for patient complexity so that physicians and other groups can compare resource utilization, complication rates, and length of stay. DRG is a system to classify hospital cases into one of originally 467 groups (Rogers, Carolin, Vaught, and Compton, 2011; Ronohardjo and Rastiko, 1982; Sachs, 2001; Sachs and Malaney, 2002). The last group (coded as 470 through v24, 999 thereafter) is considered to be "ungroupable" (Arredondo and Zúñiga, 2006;

Backer, van Roermund, Fischer, van Asseldonk, and Bergevoet, 2015; Bartsch, Hotez, Hertenstein, Diemert, Zapf, Bottazzi, and Lee, 2016). This system of classification was developed as a collaborative project by Robert B Fetter of the Yale School of Management, and John D. Thompson of the Yale School of Public Health.

The system is also referred to as "the DRGs," and its intent was to identify the "products" that a hospital provides. One example of a "product" is an appendectomy (Chen, Li, Hsieh, Chang, Lee, Lee, and Ko, 2012; Conover, Pitt, Kessler, DuBow, and Sanborn, 1995; Crump, Murdoch, and Baker, 2001). The system was developed in anticipation of convincing Congress to use it for reimbursement, to replace "cost-based" reimbursement that had been used up to that point (Daily, and Ehrlich, 1996; Deogaonkar, Hutubessy, Van Der Putten, Evers, and Jit, 2012; Dorn, 1992; Ducrotoy, Bertu, Ocholi, Gusi, Bryssinckx, Welburn, and Moriyon, 2014). DRGs are assigned by a "grouper" program based on ICD (International Classification of Diseases) diagnoses, procedures, age, sex, discharge status, and the presence of complications or comorbidities (Weycker, Edelsberg, Oster, and Tino, 2005; Wu, Perrings, Kinzig, Collins, Minteer, and Daszak, 2017; Yach, Stuckler, and Brownell, 2006). DRGs have been used in the US since 1982 to determine how much Medicare pays the hospital for each "product," since patients within each category are clinically similar and are expected to use the same level of hospital resources (Howe, Häsler, and Stärk, 2013; Howe et al., 2012). DRGs may be further grouped into Major Diagnostic Categories or MDCs. DRGs are also standard practice for establishing reimbursements for other medicare-related reimbursements such as to home healthcare providers (Foxman, 2002; Garner, Whan, Gard, and Phillips, 2001; Gayle and Hill, 2001; Gottstein, Pozio, and Nöckler, 2009).

The original objective of DRGs was to develop a classification system that identified the "products" that the patient received (Raut, 2004; Rehm, Mathers, Popova, Thavorncharoensap, Teerawattananon, and Patra, 2009; Rich and Perry, 2011). Since the introduction of DRGs in the early 1980s, the healthcare industry has evolved and developed an increased demand for a patient classification system that can serve its original objective at a higher level of sophistication and precision (Uusküla, Müürsepp, Kawai, Raag, Jürisson, and Pillsbury, 2013; Vanni, Karnon, Madan, White, Edmunds, Foss, and Legood, 2011). To meet those evolving needs, the objective of the DRG system had to expand in scope (Moné, Ibikounlé, Massougbodji, and Mouahid, 2010; Morand, 2004; Moro, Budke, Schantz, Vasquez, Santivanez, and Villavicencio, 2011). Several different DRG systems have been developed in the United States including: Medicare DRG (CMS-DRG and MS-DRG); refined DRGs (R-DRG); all patient DRGs (AP-DRG); severity DRGs (S-DRG); all patient, severity-adjusted DRGs (APS-DRG); all patient refined DRGs (APR-DRG); and the international-refined DRGs or IR-DRG (Tapia, 2003; Torgerson and Dowling, 2001; Torgerson, Carmona, and Bonifacino, 2000; Uddin Khan, Atanasova, Krueger, Ramirez, and Gray, 2013).

In health care, diagnosis codes are used as a tool to group and identify diseases, disorders, symptoms, poisonings, adverse effects of drugs and chemicals, injuries, and other reasons for patient encounters (Bergevoet, Van Schaik, Veling, Backus, and Franken, 2009; Binder, 1988; Bolos, Bacarea, and Marusteri, 2011). Diagnostic coding is the translation of written descriptions of diseases, illnesses, and injuries into codes from a particular classification (Suhrcke, Stuckler, Suk, Desai, Senek, McKee, and Rechel, 2011; Šumilo, Bormane, Asokliene, Vasilenko, Golovljova, Avsic-Zupanc, and Randolph, 2008). In medical classification, diagnosis codes are used as part of the clinical coding process alongside intervention codes (Markos and Abdela, 2016; Martin and Shepherd, 2009; McGuinness, McGlynn, Johnson, MacIntyre, Batty, Burns, and McGinty, 2012). Both diagnosis and intervention codes are assigned by a health professional trained in medical classification such as a clinical coder or Health Information Manager (Espinoza, Terashima, Herrera-Velit, and Marcos, 2010; Ezzati, Vander Hoorn, Lawes, Leach, James, Lopez, and Murray, 2005). Several diagnosis classification systems have been implemented to various degrees of success across the world (Eaton and Groopman, 2013; Eckelman, Sherman, and MacNeill, 2018; Egger, 2011; Elbe, 2007; Ernst and Hay, 1994). The various classifications have a focus towards a particular patient encounter type such as emergency, inpatient, outpatient, mental health as well as surgical care (Acemoglu and Johnson, 2007; Adda, 2016; Alloul, Sauriol, Kennedy, Laurier, Tessier, Novosel, and Contandriopoulos, 1998). The International Statistical Classification of Diseases and Related Health Problems (ICD) is one of the most widely used classification systems for diagnosis coding as it allows comparability and use of mortality and morbidity data (Amuna and Zotor, 2008; Aral, Holmes, Padian, and Cates, 1996; Arbabi, Nezami, Hooshyar, and Delavari, 2018). These codes can be particularly useful when managing a major pandemic because they not only track case and severity; but also potentially identify the resources that are required to manage patients effectively (Peckham, 2013; Perrings et al., 2002, 2014).

CHAPTER 4 SUMMARY

The typologies of disease epidemicsDisease epidemics are not set in stone, not least because of the complexity and diversity of the underlying phenomena itself. However, epidemics have been generally classified according to their causes, impact, transmission, time or geographical location, and severity. In the next chapter, we further explore the modalities of these disease epidemicsDisease epidemics, a topic that has already been briefly introduced in Chapter 4.

Chapter 5

Outbreak Modalities of Disease Epidemics Disease Epidemics

CONTENTS

The modalities of a disease outbreak are important to health planners and responders because they implicitly tell us about the underlying causes and how the disease actually arises. In this chapter, we explore these modalities in terms of common sources, propagated outbreaks, contagion, artificial or synthetic diseases, and the role of population profiles, including genetics. By the end of this chapter, the reader should have a good idea of how the modalities of disease outbreaks are classified and analyzed.

5.1. COMMON SOURCE DISEASE OUTBREAKS

In epidemiology, an outbreak is a sudden increase in occurrences of a disease in a particular time and place (Borghol, Suderman, McArdle, Racine, Hallett, Pembrey, and Szyf, 2012; Brandes, 2008; Brown, Lipscomb, and Snyder, 2001). It may affect a small and localized group or impact upon thousands of people across an entire continent (Bwire, Munier, Ouedraogo, Heyerdahl, Komakech, Kagirita, and Makumbi, 2017; Canali, Aragrande, Angheben, Capelli, Drigo, Gobbi, and Cassini, 2020). Four linked cases of a rare infectious disease may be sufficient to constitute an outbreak (Armelagos, Brown, and Turner, 2005; Arokiasamy and Krishnan, 1994; Arora, 2001, 2005; Arredondo and Zúñiga, 2004). Outbreaks include epidemics, which term is normally only used for infectious diseases, as well as diseases with an environmental origin, such as water or foodborne disease (Oleś, Gudowska-Nowak, and Kleczkowski, 2012; Otte, Nugent, and McLeod, 2004; Ozawa, Portnoy, Getaneh, Clark, Knoll, Bishai, and Patwardhan, 2016). They may affect a region in a country or a group of countries (Bonds, Keenan, Rohani, and Sachs, 2010; Boni, Galvani, Wickelgren, and Malani, 2013; Bonovas and Nikolopoulos, 2012). Pandemics are near-global disease outbreaks when multiple countries across the world are infected (Kim and Goldie, 2008; Klein, Laxminarayan, Smith, and Gilligan, 2007; Klepac, Laxminarayan, and Grenfell, 2011). The outbreak may be mapped through Bayesian prediction (see Figure 5.1, for an example).

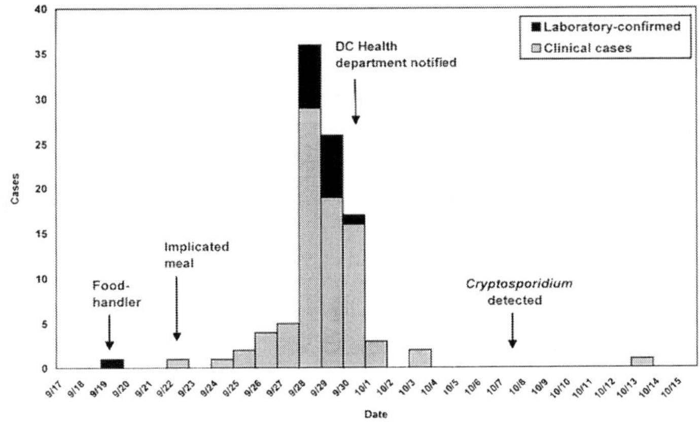

Figure 5.1. Example of a Bayesian prediction of a disease outbreak.

Source: Science Direct.

The terms "outbreak" and "epidemic" have often been used interchangeably (St George, 1986; Steben and Duarte-Franco, 2007; Stehr-Green and Schantz, 1987; Stuckler, 2008; Stuckler and Siegel, 2011). Researchers Manfred S. Green and colleagues propose that the latter term be restricted to larger events, pointing out that Chambers Concise Dictionary and Stedman's Medical Dictionary acknowledge this distinction (Poundstone, Strathdee, and Celentano, 2004; Pritchett, Thilmany, and Johnson, 2005; Pugliatti, Beghi, Forsgren, Ekman, and Sobocki, 2007). When investigating disease outbreaks, the epidemiology profession has developed a number of widely accepted steps (Casamassimo, Thikkurissy, Edelstein, and Maiorini, 2009; Castro, Wilson, and Bloom, 2017). As described by the United States Centers for Disease Control and Prevention (CDC), these include a number of steps (Yi-Xin and Manderson, 2005; Zadoks, 2008; Zhan, Li, Wang, Sun, Geng, Xiong, and de Hoog, 2015; Zhang, Song, Cai, and Zhou, 2008). First, identify the existence of the outbreak. Second, verify the diagnosis related to the outbreak (Weycker, Edelsberg, Oster, and Tino, 2005; Wu, Perrings, Kinzig, Collins, Minteer, and Daszak, 2017; Yach, Stuckler, and Brownell, 2006). Third, create a case definition to define who or what is included as a case (Uusküla, Müürsepp, Kawai, Raag, Jürisson, and Pillsbury, 2013; Vanni, Karnon, Madan, White, Edmunds, Foss, and Legood, 2011). Fourth, map the spread of the outbreak using Information technology as diagnosis is reported to insurance (Tapia, 2003; Torgerson and Dowling, 2001; Torgerson, Carmona, and Bonifacino, 2000; Uddin Khan, Atanasova, Krueger, Ramirez, and Gray, 2013). Fifth, develop a hypothesis in terms of what appears to be causing the outbreak (Suhrcke, Stuckler, Suk, Desai, Senek, McKee, and Rechel, 2011; Šumilo, Bormane, Asokliene, Vasilenko, Golovljova, Avsic-Zupanc, and Randolph, 2008). Fifth, style the hypotheses through data collection and analysis (St George, 1986; Steben and Duarte-Franco, 2007; Stehr-Green and Schantz, 1987; Stuckler, 2008; Stuckler and Siegel, 2011). Then you refine the hypothesis and carry out further study (Saleha, 1991; Sibert, Rigaud, Delavierre, and Labat, 2010; Skrepnek and Skrepnek, 2004; Sloane, 2009; Sockett, 1993). This is followed by the development and implementation of control and prevention systems (Rogers, Carolin, Vaught, and Compton, 2011; Ronohardjo and Rastiko, 1982; Sachs, 2001; Sachs and Malaney, 2002). Lastly, you release the findings to the greater communities (Raut, 2004; Rehm, Mathers, Popova, Thavorncharoensap, Teerawattananon, and Patra, 2009; Rich and Perry, 2011).

The order of the above steps and relative amount of effort and resources used in each varies from outbreak to outbreak (Purevdawa, Moon, Baigalmaa, Davaajav, Smith, and Vermund, 1997; Ramesh, Malla, Raju, Sehgal, Ganguly, Mahajan, and Dilawari, 1990). For example, prevention and control measures are usually implemented very early in the investigation, often before the causative agent is known (Poundstone, Strathdee, and Celentano, 2004; Pritchett, Thilmany, and Johnson, 2005; Pugliatti, Beghi, Forsgren, Ekman, and Sobocki, 2007). In many situations, promoting good hygiene and hand-washing is one of the first things recommended (Perry and Randolph, 1999; Philipson, 2000; Philipson and Posner, 1996; Pongchaiyakul, Songpattanasilp, and Taechakraichana, 2008). Other interventions may be added as the investigation moves forward and more information is obtained (Peckham, 2013; Perrings et al., 2002, 2014). Waiting until the end of an investigation to implement prevention and control measures is a sure way to lose one's job (Pal, Kerorsa, Marami, and Kandi, 2020; Paterson, Otte, Slingenbergh, Wint, and Rogers, 2000; Pearce and Merletti, 2006). In outbreaks identified through notifiable disease surveillance, reports are often linked to laboratory results and verifying the diagnosis is straight forward (Ozmen, Kurşun, and Ozcelik, 2005; Paarlberg, Hillberg, Lee, and Mathews, 2008; Paisley, Vraa-Andersen, Dybkjaer, Møller, Christensen, Mousing, and Agger, 1993). In outbreaks of unknown etiology, determining, and verifying the diagnosis can be a significant part of the investigation with respect to time and resources (Oleś, Gudowska-Nowak, and Kleczkowski, 2012; Otte, Nugent, and McLeod, 2004; Ozawa, Portnoy, Getaneh, Clark, Knoll, Bishai, and Patwardhan, 2016). Several steps are usually going on at any point in time during the investigation (Narrod, Zinsstag, and Tiongco, 2012; Nascimento and de Oliveira, 2014; O'Brien, Lahue, Caro, and Davidson, 2007). Steps may be repeated (Moné, Ibikounlé, Massougbodji, and Mouahid, 2010; Morand, 2004; Moro, Budke, Schantz, Vasquez, Santivanez, and Villavicencio, 2011). For example, initial case definitions are often established to be intentionally broad but later refined as more is learned about the outbreak (Markos and Abdela, 2016; Martin and Shepherd, 2009; McGuinness, McGlynn, Johnson, MacIntyre, Batty, Burns, and McGinty, 2012). The above list has nine steps, others have more. Implementing active surveillance to identify additional cases is often added (Krieger, 2001a, b; Lemma, 1969; Liu, Maniadakis, Gray, and Rayner, 2002; López, Torné, Franco, San-Martin, Viayna, Barrull, and Perulero, 2018).

Outbreak debriefing and review has also been recognized as an additional final step and iterative process by the Public Health Agency of Canada (Kim and Goldie, 2008; Klein, Laxminarayan, Smith, and Gilligan, 2007; Klepac, Laxminarayan, and Grenfell, 2011). There are several outbreak patterns, which can be useful in identifying the transmission method or source, and predicting the future rate of infection (Jenkins, Baingana, Ahmad, McDaid, and Atun, 2011; Johnson, Alvarez-Pasquin, Bijl, Franco, Gaillat, Clara, and Weinke, 2015). Each has a distinctive epidemic curve, or histogram of case infections and deaths (Howe, Häsler, and Stärk, 2013; Howe et al., 2012). Outbreaks can be categorized by the way that the causative agent (usually a microorganism) is spread within the population to reach new susceptible people (Hart and Halden, 2020; Häsler, Howe, and Stärk, 2011; Henschke, Kamper, and Maher, 2015; Hochberg, 1992). The place (or object) where people get infected by the microorganism is called 'the source' of the outbreak (Foxman, 2002; Garner, Whan, Gard, and Phillips, 2001; Gayle and Hill, 2001; Gottstein, Pozio, and Nöckler, 2009).

When all (or most) cases in an outbreak are infected by the same source, then we call such an outbreak a common source outbreak (Fenichel, 2013; Fenichel et al., 2011; Fogel, 1994). Common source outbreaks where the source has infected cases at one particular geographical location, during a short period of time, are called 'point source outbreaks' (Espinoza, Terashima, Herrera-Velit, and Marcos, 2010; Ezzati, Vander Hoorn, Lawes, Leach, James, Lopez, and Murray, 2005). In such situations, the source is said to be located 'at a single point in time and place' (Eaton and Groopman, 2013; Eckelman, Sherman, and MacNeill, 2018; Egger, 2011; Elbe, 2007; Ernst and Hay, 1994). These outbreaks have a typical bell-shaped epidemic curve, that increases sharply, peaks, and then decline sharply, which reflects the normal distribution of the incubation period of the causative agent in humans (Daily, and Ehrlich, 1996; Deogaonkar, Hutubessy, Van Der Putten, Evers, and Jit, 2012; Dorn, 1992; Ducrotoy, Bertu, Ocholi, Gusi, Bryssinckx, Welburn, and Moriyon, 2014). For this reason, the epidemic curve of a point source outbreak can help us identify the moment of transmission, that is to say, when all cases have been exposed to the source). The next section explores propagated disease outbreaks.

5.2. PROPAGATED DISEASE OUTBREAKS

Propagated disease outbreaks occur when transmission occurs from person to person (Chen, Li, Hsieh, Chang, Lee, Lee, and Ko, 2012; Conover, Pitt, Kessler, DuBow, and Sanborn, 1995; Crump, Murdoch, and Baker, 2001). A contagious disease is a subset category of transmissible diseases, which are transmitted to other persons, either by physical contact with the person suffering the disease (Bwire, Munier, Ouedraogo, Heyerdahl, Komakech, Kagirita, and Makumbi, 2017; Canali, Aragrande, Angheben, Capelli, Drigo, Gobbi, and Cassini, 2020). It can be by casual contact with their secretions or objects touched by them or airborne route among other routes (Casamassimo, Thikkurissy, Edelstein, and Maiorini, 2009; Castro, Wilson, and Bloom, 2017). Contagiousness varies between diseases (Buckley, 1984; Budke, Jiamin, Qian, and Torgerson, 2005; Bundy, Arámbulo III, and Grey, 1983; Buzby and Roberts, 2009). Non-contagious infections, by contrast, usually require a special mode of transmission between persons or hosts (Borghol, Suderman, McArdle, Racine, Hallett, Pembrey, and Szyf, 2012; Brandes, 2008; Brown, Lipscomb, and Snyder, 2001). There are several factors that can contribute to the transmission of disease, including climate change, demographic changes, and urbanization (see Figure 5.2).

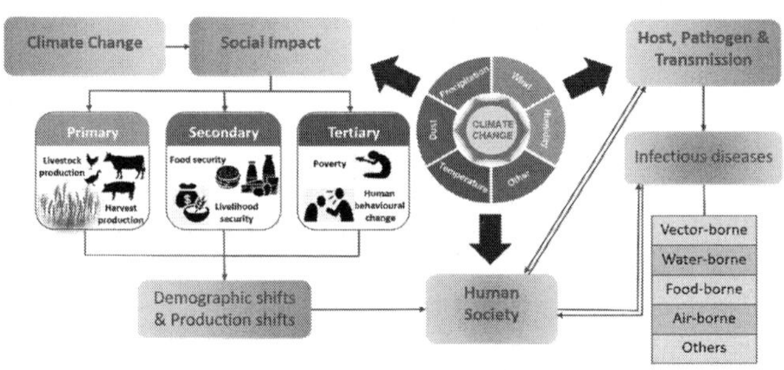

Figure 5.2. Factors the aggravate disease transmission.

Source: MDPI.

These include need for intermediate vector species (mosquitoes that carry malaria) or by non-casual transfer of bodily fluid such as transfusions, needle sharing or sexual contact (Bonds, Keenan, Rohani, and Sachs, 2010; Boni, Galvani, Wickelgren, and Malani, 2013; Bonovas and Nikolopoulos, 2012). The boundary between contagious and non-contagious infectious diseases is not perfectly drawn, as illustrated classically by tuberculosis, which is clearly transmissible from person to person, but was not classically considered a contagious disease (Bergevoet, Van Schaik, Veling, Backus, and Franken, 2009; Binder, 1988; Bolos, Bacarea, and Marusteri, 2011). In the present day, most sexually transmitted infections are considered contagious, but only some of them are subject to medical isolation (Bausch and Schwarz, 2014; Bausch et al., 2001; Benner, Carabin, Sánchez-Serrano, Budke, and Carmena, 2010).

A disease may be known to be contagious, but its causative factors remain undetermined. A contagion may be more infectious if the incubation period is long (Arredondo and Zúñiga, 2006; Backer, van Roermund, Fischer, van Asseldonk, and Bergevoet, 2015; Bartsch, Hotez, Hertenstein, Diemert, Zapf, Bottazzi, and Lee, 2016). Historical meaning Originally, the term referred to a contagion (a derivative of 'contact') or disease transmissible only by direct physical contact (Armelagos, Brown, and Turner, 2005; Arokiasamy and Krishnan, 1994; Arora, 2001, 2005; Arredondo and Zúñiga, 2004). In the modern-day, the term has sometimes been broadened to encompass any communicable or infectious disease (Amuna and Zotor, 2008; Aral, Holmes, Padian, and Cates, 1996; Arbabi, Nezami, Hooshyar, and Delavari, 2018). Often the word can only be understood in context, where it is used to emphasize very infectious, easily transmitted, or especially severe communicable disease (Acemoglu and Johnson, 2007; Adda, 2016; Alloul, Sauriol, Kennedy, Laurier, Tessier, Novosel, and Contandriopoulos, 1998). Most epidemics are caused by contagious diseases, with occasional exceptions, such as yellow fever (Abegunde and Stanciole, 2008; Abramowitz, Lacau Saint Guily, Moyal-Barracco, Bergeron, Borne, Dahlab, and Bénard, 2018). The spread of non-contagious communicable diseases is changed either very little or not at all by medical isolation of ill persons or medical quarantine for exposed persons (Ozmen, Kurşun, and Ozcelik, 2005; Paarlberg, Hillberg, Lee, and Mathews, 2008; Paisley, Vraa-Andersen, Dybkjaer, Møller, Christensen, Mousing, and Agger, 1993). Thus, a "contagious disease" is sometimes defined in practical terms, as a disease for which isolation or quarantine are useful public health responses

(Bonds, Keenan, Rohani, and Sachs, 2010; Boni, Galvani, Wickelgren, and Malani, 2013; Bonovas and Nikolopoulos, 2012).

Some locations are better suited for the research into the contagious pathogens due to the reduced risk of transmission afforded by a remote or isolated location (Espinoza, Terashima, Herrera-Velit, and Marcos, 2010; Ezzati, Vander Hoorn, Lawes, Leach, James, Lopez, and Murray, 2005). Negative room pressure is a technique in health care facilities based on aerobiological designs (Buckley, 1984; Budke, Jiamin, Qian, and Torgerson, 2005; Bundy, Arámbulo III, and Grey, 1983; Buzby and Roberts, 2009). An asymptomatic carrier (healthy carrier or just carrier) is a person or other organism that has become infected with a pathogen, but that displays no signs or symptoms (Bwire, Munier, Ouedraogo, Heyerdahl, Komakech, Kagirita, and Makumbi, 2017; Canali, Aragrande, Angheben, Capelli, Drigo, Gobbi, and Cassini, 2020). Although unaffected by the pathogen, carriers can transmit it to others or develop symptoms in later stages of the disease (Yi-Xin and Manderson, 2005; Zadoks, 2008; Zhan, Li, Wang, Sun, Geng, Xiong, and de Hoog, 2015; Zhang, Song, Cai, and Zhou, 2008). Asymptomatic carriers play a critical role in the transmission of common infectious diseases such as typhoid, HIV, C. difficile, influenzas, cholera, tuberculosis, and COVID-19 (Pal, Kerorsa, Marami, and Kandi, 2020; Paterson, Otte, Slingenbergh, Wint, and Rogers, 2000; Pearce and Merletti, 2006). Specifically, the latter is often associated with "robust T-cell immunity" in more than a quarter of patients studied (Canali, Aragrande, Angheben, Capelli, Drigo, Gobbi, and Cassini, 2020). While the mechanism of disease-carrying is still unknown, researchers have made progress towards understanding how certain pathogens can remain dormant in a human for a period of time (Pal, Kerorsa, Marami, and Kandi, 2020; Paterson, Otte, Slingenbergh, Wint, and Rogers, 2000; Pearce and Merletti, 2006). A better understanding of asymptomatic disease carriers is crucial to the fields of medicine and public health as they work towards mitigating the spread of common infectious diseases (Jenkins, Baingana, Ahmad, McDaid, and Atun, 2011; Johnson, Alvarez-Pasquin, Bijl, Franco, Gaillat, Clara, and Weinke, 2015).

Asymptomatic carriers can be categorized by their current disease state (Abegunde and Stanciole, 2008; Abramowitz, Lacau Saint Guily, Moyal-Barracco, Bergeron, Borne, Dahlab, and Bénard, 2018). When an individual transmits pathogens immediately the following infection but prior to developing symptoms, they are known as an incubatory carrier (Kim and Goldie, 2008; Klein, Laxminarayan, Smith, and Gilligan, 2007;

Klepac, Laxminarayan, and Grenfell, 2011). Humans are also capable of spreading disease following a period of illness (Chen, Li, Hsieh, Chang, Lee, Lee, and Ko, 2012; Conover, Pitt, Kessler, DuBow, and Sanborn, 1995; Crump, Murdoch, and Baker, 2001). Typically thinking themselves cured of the disease, these individuals are known as convalescent carriers (Weycker, Edelsberg, Oster, and Tino, 2005; Wu, Perrings, Kinzig, Collins, Minteer, and Daszak, 2017; Yach, Stuckler, and Brownell, 2006). Viral diseases such as hepatitis and poliomyelitis are frequently transmitted in this manner (Perry and Randolph, 1999; Philipson, 2000; Philipson and Posner, 1996; Pongchaiyakul, Songpattanasilp, and Taechakraichana, 2008). "Healthy carriers" never exhibit signs or symptoms of the disease, yet are capable of infecting others, and are often considered to be the "classic" asymptomatic carriers (Uusküla, Müürsepp, Kawai, Raag, Jürisson, and Pillsbury, 2013; Vanni, Karnon, Madan, White, Edmunds, Foss, and Legood, 2011). The limited information on the prevalence of asymptomatic carriers creates a considerable difficulty when planning public health initiatives (St George, 1986; Steben and Duarte-Franco, 2007; Stehr-Green and Schantz, 1987; Stuckler, 2008; Stuckler and Siegel, 2011). Given that disease surveillance is dependent on estimates for both the asymptomatic rates and symptomatic rates of disease, the lack of information on the prevalence of carriers can lead to insufficient initiatives for the mitigation of common public health concerns such as C. difficile or influenza (Acemoglu and Johnson, 2007; Adda, 2016; Alloul, Sauriol, Kennedy, Laurier, Tessier, Novosel, and Contandriopoulos, 1998). The next section of this chapter focuses on non-contagious disease outbreaks.

5.3. NON-CONTAGIOUS DISEASE OUTBREAKS

A non-communicable disease (or NCD) is a disease that is not transmissible directly from one person to another. NCDs include Parkinson's disease, autoimmune diseases, strokes, most heart diseases, most cancers, diabetes, chronic kidney disease, osteoarthritis, osteoporosis, Alzheimer's disease, cataracts, and others (Amuna and Zotor, 2008; Aral, Holmes, Padian, and Cates, 1996; Arbabi, Nezami, Hooshyar, and Delavari, 2018). NCDs may be chronic or acute (Krieger, 2001a, b; Lemma, 1969; Liu, Maniadakis, Gray, and Rayner, 2002; López, Torné, Franco, San-Martin, Viayna, Barrull, and Perulero, 2018). Most are non-infectious, although there are some non-communicable infectious diseases (Armelagos, Brown, and Turner, 2005; Arokiasamy and Krishnan, 1994; Arora, 2001, 2005; Arredondo and Zúñiga,

2004). Examples include parasitic diseases in which the parasite's life cycle does not include direct host-to-host transmission (Poundstone, Strathdee, and Celentano, 2004; Pritchett, Thilmany, and Johnson, 2005; Pugliatti, Beghi, Forsgren, Ekman, and Sobocki, 2007). NCDs are the leading cause of death globally. In 2012, they caused 68% of all deaths (38 million) up from 60% in 2000 (Suhrcke, Stuckler, Suk, Desai, Senek, McKee, and Rechel, 2011; Šumilo, Bormane, Asokliene, Vasilenko, Golovljova, Avsic-Zupanc, and Randolph, 2008). About half were under age 70 and half were women.

Risk factors such as a person's background, lifestyle, and environment increase the likelihood of certain NCDs (Bergevoet, Van Schaik, Veling, Backus, and Franken, 2009; Binder, 1988; Bolos, Bacarea, and Marusteri, 2011). Every year, at least 5 million people die because of tobacco use and about 2.8 million die from being overweight (Arredondo and Zúñiga, 2006; Backer, van Roermund, Fischer, van Asseldonk, and Bergevoet, 2015; Bartsch, Hotez, Hertenstein, Diemert, Zapf, Bottazzi, and Lee, 2016). High cholesterol accounts for roughly 2.6 million deaths and 7.5 million dies because of high blood pressure (Howe, Häsler, and Stärk, 2013; Howe et al., 2012). Some nations have voluntarily agreed to certain targets for 2025 when dealing with NCDs (see Figure 5.3).

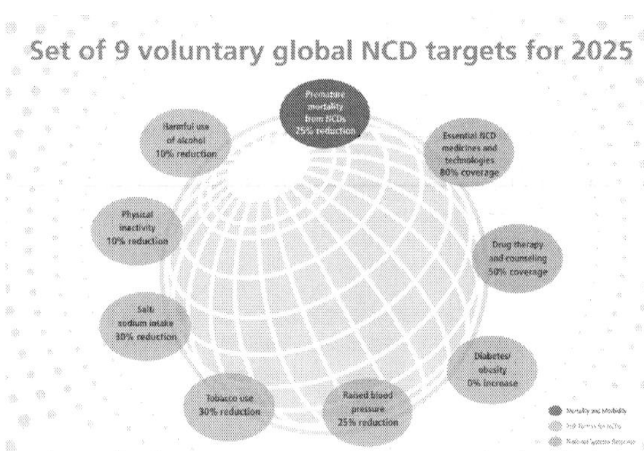

Figure 5.3. Targets for non-communicable diseases by 2025.

Source: Physiopedia.

Risk factors such as a person's background, lifestyle and environment are known to increase the likelihood of certain non-communicable diseases (Raut, 2004; Rehm, Mathers, Popova, Thavorncharoensap, Teerawattananon, and Patra, 2009; Rich and Perry, 2011). They include age, gender, genetics, exposure to air pollution, and behaviors such as smoking, unhealthy diet and physical inactivity which can lead to hypertension and obesity, in turn leading to increased risk of many NCDs (Hart and Halden, 2020; Häsler, Howe, and Stärk, 2011; Henschke, Kamper, and Maher, 2015; Hochberg, 1992). Most NCDs are considered preventable because they are caused by modifiable risk factors (Markos and Abdela, 2016; Martin and Shepherd, 2009; McGuinness, McGlynn, Johnson, MacIntyre, Batty, Burns, and McGinty, 2012). The WHO's World Health Report 2002 identified five important risk factors for non-communicable disease in the top 10 leading risks to health (Foxman, 2002; Garner, Whan, Gard, and Phillips, 2001; Gayle and Hill, 2001; Gottstein, Pozio, and Nöckler, 2009). These are raised blood pressure, raised cholesterol, tobacco use, alcohol consumption, and being overweight (Moné, Ibikounlé, Massougbodji, and Mouahid, 2010; Morand, 2004; Moro, Budke, Schantz, Vasquez, Santivanez, and Villavicencio, 2011). The other factors associated with higher risk of NCDs include a person's economic and social conditions, also known as the social determinants of health (Eaton and Groopman, 2013; Eckelman, Sherman, and MacNeill, 2018; Egger, 2011; Elbe, 2007; Ernst and Hay, 1994).

It has been estimated that if the primary risk factors were eliminated, 80% of the cases of heart disease, stroke, and type 2 diabetes and 40% of cancers could be prevented (Oleś, Gudowska-Nowak, and Kleczkowski, 2012; Otte, Nugent, and McLeod, 2004; Ozawa, Portnoy, Getaneh, Clark, Knoll, Bishai, and Patwardhan, 2016). Interventions targeting the main risk factors could have a significant impact on reducing the burden of disease worldwide (Rogers, Carolin, Vaught, and Compton, 2011; Ronohardjo and Rastiko, 1982; Sachs, 2001; Sachs and Malaney, 2002). Efforts focused on better diet and increased physical activity have been shown to control the prevalence of NCDs (Bausch and Schwarz, 2014; Bausch et al., 2001; Benner, Carabin, Sánchez-Serrano, Budke, and Carmena, 2010). NCDs include many environmental diseases covering a broad category of avoidable and unavoidable human health conditions caused by external factors, such as sunlight, nutrition, pollution, and lifestyle choices (Purevdawa, Moon, Baigalmaa, Davaajav, Smith, and Vermund, 1997; Ramesh, Malla, Raju, Sehgal, Ganguly, Mahajan, and Dilawari, 1990). The diseases of affluence are non-infectious diseases with environmental causes (Borghol, Suderman, McArdle, Racine, Hallett, Pembrey, and Szyf, 2012; Brandes, 2008; Brown, Lipscomb, and Snyder, 2001). Examples include: many types of cardiovascular disease (CVD); chronic obstructive pulmonary disease

(COPD) caused by smoking tobacco; diabetes mellitus type 2; lower back pain caused by too little exercise; malnutrition caused by too little food, or eating the wrong kinds of food (e.g., scurvy from lack of Vitamin C); skin cancer caused by radiation from the sun; and obesity (Tapia, 2003; Torgerson and Dowling, 2001; Torgerson, Carmona, and Bonifacino, 2000; Uddin Khan, Atanasova, Krueger, Ramirez, and Gray, 2013).

Genetic disorders are caused by errors in genetic information that produce diseases in the affected people (Saleha, 1991; Sibert, Rigaud, Delavierre, and Labat, 2010; Skrepnek and Skrepnek, 2004; Sloane, 2009; Sockett, 1993). The origin of these genetic errors may include spontaneous errors or mutations to the genome; a change in chromosome numbers, such as Down syndrome; a defect in a gene caused by mutation, such as Cystic fibrosis; or an increase in the amount of genetic information, such as Chimerism or Heterochromia (Peckham, 2013; Perrings et al., 2002, 2014). Cystic fibrosis is an example of an inherited disease that is caused by a mutation on a gene (Daily, and Ehrlich, 1996; Deogaonkar, Hutubessy, Van Der Putten, Evers, and Jit, 2012; Dorn, 1992; Ducrotoy, Bertu, Ocholi, Gusi, Bryssinckx, Welburn, and Moriyon, 2014). The faulty gene impairs the normal movement of sodium chloride in and out of cells, which causes the mucus-secreting organs to produce abnormally thick mucus (Fenichel, 2013; Fenichel et al., 2011; Fogel, 1994). The gene is recessive, meaning that a person must have two copies of the faulty gene for them to develop the disease (Narrod, Zinsstag, and Tiongco, 2012; Nascimento and de Oliveira, 2014; O'Brien, Lahue, Caro, and Davidson, 2007). Cystic fibrosis affects the respiratory, digestive, and reproductive systems, as well as the sweat glands (Casamassimo, Thikkurissy, Edelstein, and Maiorini, 2009; Castro, Wilson, and Bloom, 2017). The mucus secreted is very thick and blocks passageways in the lungs and digestive tracts (Abegunde and Stanciole, 2008; Abramowitz, Lacau Saint Guily, Moyal-Barracco, Bergeron, Borne, Dahlab, and Bénard, 2018). This mucus causes problems with breathing and with the digestion and absorption of nutrients (Acemoglu and Johnson, 2007; Adda, 2016; Alloul, Sauriol, Kennedy, Laurier, Tessier, Novosel, and Contandriopoulos, 1998).

Historically, many NCDs were associated with economic development and were so-called a "diseases of the rich" (Amuna and Zotor, 2008; Aral, Holmes, Padian, and Cates, 1996; Arbabi, Nezami, Hooshyar, and Delavari, 2018). The burden of non-communicable diseases in developing countries has increased, however, with an estimated 80% of the four main types of NCDs including CVDs, cancers, chronic respiratory diseases and diabetes

(Armelagos, Brown, and Turner, 2005; Arokiasamy and Krishnan, 1994; Arora, 2001, 2005; Arredondo and Zúñiga, 2004). These are now occurring in low and middle-income countries. Action Plan for the Global Strategy for the Prevention and Control of non-communicable Diseases and with two-thirds of people who are affected by diabetes now residing in developing nations, NCD can no longer be considered just a problem affecting affluent estimation of the economic impact of chronic non-communicable diseases in selected countries (Arredondo and Zúñiga, 2006; Backer, van Roermund, Fischer, van Asseldonk, and Bergevoet, 2015; Bartsch, Hotez, Hertenstein, Diemert, Zapf, Bottazzi, and Lee, 2016). According to a new World Health Organization (WHO) report: deaths from non-communicable diseases are on the rise, with developing world hit hardest (Bausch and Schwarz, 2014; Bausch et al., 2001; Benner, Carabin, Sánchez-Serrano, Budke, and Carmena, 2010). As previously stated, in 2008 alone, NCD's were the cause of 63% of deaths worldwide; a number that is expected to rise considerably in the near future if measures are not taken (Bergevoet, Van Schaik, Veling, Backus, and Franken, 2009; Binder, 1988; Bolos, Bacarea, and Marusteri, 2011).

If present growth trends are maintained, by 2020, NCDs will attribute to 7 out of every 10 deaths in developing countries (Bonds, Keenan, Rohani, and Sachs, 2010; Boni, Galvani, Wickelgren, and Malani, 2013; Bonovas and Nikolopoulos, 2012). It is expected that NCDs will be responsible for killing 52 million people annually worldwide by 2030 (Borghol, Suderman, McArdle, Racine, Hallett, Pembrey, and Szyf, 2012; Brandes, 2008; Brown, Lipscomb, and Snyder, 2001). With statistics such as these, it comes as no surprise that international entities such as the WHO and World Bank Human Development Network have identified the prevention and control of NCDs as an increasingly important discussion item on the global health agenda (Buckley, 1984; Budke, Jiamin, Qian, and Torgerson, 2005; Bundy, Arámbulo III, and Grey, 1983; Buzby and Roberts, 2009). Thus, should policymakers and communities mobilize "and make prevention and targeted treatment of such diseases a priority (Bwire, Munier, Ouedraogo, Heyerdahl, Komakech, Kagirita, and Makumbi, 2017; Canali, Aragrande, Angheben, Capelli, Drigo, Gobbi, and Cassini, 2020). Some of the recommended measures include reducing the levels of salt in foods, limiting inappropriate marketing of unhealthy foods and non-alcoholic beverages to children, imposing controls on harmful alcohol use, raising taxes on tobacco, and legislating to curb smoking in public places (Casamassimo, Thikkurissy, Edelstein, and Maiorini, 2009; Castro, Wilson, and Bloom, 2017). The next section considers the possibilities of manufactured or synthetic disease epidemicsDisease epidemics, a topic that was touched on in previous chapters with reference to biowarfare.

5.4. MANUFACTURED OR ARTIFICIAL DISEASE OUTBREAKS

Synthetic virology is a branch of virology engaged in the study and engineering of synthetic man-made viruses (Casamassimo, Thikkurissy, Edelstein, and Maiorini, 2009; Castro, Wilson, and Bloom, 2017). It is a multidisciplinary research field at the intersection of virology, synthetic biology, computational biology, and DNA nanotechnology, from which it borrows and integrates its concepts and methodologies (Chen, Li, Hsieh, Chang, Lee, Lee, and Ko, 2012; Conover, Pitt, Kessler, DuBow, and Sanborn, 1995; Crump, Murdoch, and Baker, 2001). There is a wide range of applications for synthetic viral technology such as medical treatments, investigative tools, and reviving organisms (Daily, and Ehrlich, 1996; Deogaonkar, Hutubessy, Van Der Putten, Evers, and Jit, 2012; Dorn, 1992; Ducrotoy, Bertu, Ocholi, Gusi, Bryssinckx, Welburn, and Moriyon, 2014).

Advances in genome sequencing technology and oligonucleotide synthesis paved the way for the construction of synthetic genomes based on previously sequenced genomes (Eaton and Groopman, 2013; Eckelman, Sherman, and MacNeill, 2018; Egger, 2011; Elbe, 2007; Ernst and Hay, 1994). Both RNA and DNA viruses can be made using existing methods (Espinoza, Terashima, Herrera-Velit, and Marcos, 2010; Ezzati, Vander Hoorn, Lawes, Leach, James, Lopez, and Murray, 2005). RNA viruses have historically been utilized due to the typically small genome size and existing reverse transcription machinery present (Fenichel, 2013; Fenichel et al., 2011; Fogel, 1994). Figure 5.4 highlights the possibility of physical, chemical, and synthetic virology.

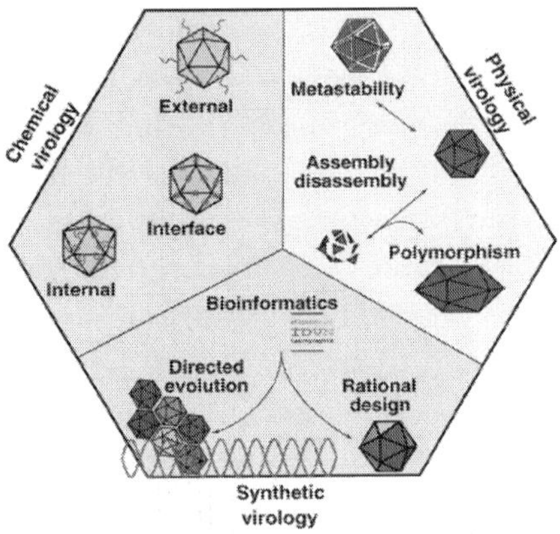

Figure 5.4. Physical, synthetic, and chemical virology.

Source: Wiley Online Library.

The first man-made infectious viruses generated without any natural template were of the poliovirus and the φX174 bacteriophage (Foxman, 2002; Garner, Whan, Gard, and Phillips, 2001; Gayle and Hill, 2001; Gottstein, Pozio, and Nöckler, 2009). With synthetic live viruses, it is not whole viruses that are synthesized but rather their genome at first, both in the case of DNA and RNA viruses (Hart and Halden, 2020; Häsler, Howe, and Stärk, 2011; Henschke, Kamper, and Maher, 2015; Hochberg, 1992). For many viruses, viral RNA is infectious when introduced into a cell (during infection or after reverse transcription). These organisms are able to sustain an infectious life cycle upon introduction in vivo (Howe, Häsler, and Stärk, 2013; Howe et al., 2012). This technology is now being used to investigate novel vaccine strategies (Jenkins, Baingana, Ahmad, McDaid, and Atun, 2011; Johnson, Alvarez-Pasquin, Bijl, Franco, Gaillat, Clara, and Weinke, 2015). The ability to synthesize viruses has far-reaching consequences, since viruses can no longer be regarded as extinct, as long as the information of their genome sequence is known and permissive cells are available (Kim and Goldie, 2008; Klein, Laxminarayan, Smith, and Gilligan, 2007; Klepac, Laxminarayan, and Grenfell, 2011). By 2020, the full-length genome sequences of 9,240 different viruses, including the smallpox virus, are publicly available in an online database maintained by the National Institutes of Health (Krieger, 2001a, b; Lemma, 1969; Liu, Maniadakis, Gray, and Rayner, 2002; López, Torné, Franco, San-Martin, Viayna, Barrull, and Perulero, 2018). Synthetic viruses have also been researched as potential gene therapy tools (Markos and Abdela, 2016; Martin and Shepherd, 2009; McGuinness, McGlynn,

Johnson, MacIntyre, Batty, Burns, and McGinty, 2012). Bioterrorism is terrorism involving the intentional release or dissemination of biological agents (Moné, Ibikounlé, Massougbodji, and Mouahid, 2010; Morand, 2004; Moro, Budke, Schantz, Vasquez, Santivanez, and Villavicencio, 2011). These agents are bacteria, viruses, insects, fungi, or toxins, and maybe in a naturally occurring or a human-modified form, in much the same way in biological warfare (Narrod, Zinsstag, and Tiongco, 2012; Nascimento and de Oliveira, 2014; O'Brien, Lahue, Caro, and Davidson, 2007). Further, modern agribusiness is vulnerable to anti-agricultural attacks by terrorists, and such attacks can seriously damage the economy as well as consumer confidence (Oleś, Gudowska-Nowak, and Kleczkowski, 2012; Otte, Nugent, and McLeod, 2004; Ozawa, Portnoy, Getaneh, Clark, Knoll, Bishai, and Patwardhan, 2016). The later destructive activity is called agrobioterrorism and is subtype of agro-terrorism (Ozmen, Kurşun, and Ozcelik, 2005; Paarlberg, Hillberg, Lee, and Mathews, 2008; Paisley, Vraa-Andersen, Dybkjaer, Møller, Christensen, Mousing, and Agger, 1993). Bioterrorism is the deliberate release of viruses, bacteria, toxins or other harmful agents to cause illness or death in people, animals, or plants (Pal, Kerorsa, Marami, and Kandi, 2020; Paterson, Otte, Slingenbergh, Wint, and Rogers, 2000; Pearce and Merletti, 2006). These agents are typically found in nature but could be mutated or altered to increase their ability to cause disease, make them resistant to current medicines, or to increase their ability to be spread into the environment (Peckham, 2013; Perrings et al., 2002, 2014). Biological agents can be spread through the air, water, or in food (Perry and Randolph, 1999; Philipson, 2000; Philipson and Posner, 1996; Pongchaiyakul, Songpattanasilp, and Taechakraichana, 2008). Biological agents are attractive to terrorists because they are extremely difficult to detect and do not cause illness for several hours to several days (Poundstone, Strathdee, and Celentano, 2004; Pritchett, Thilmany, and Johnson, 2005; Pugliatti, Beghi, Forsgren, Ekman, and Sobocki, 2007).

Some bioterrorism agents, like the smallpox virus, can be spread from person to person and some, like anthrax, cannot be easily spread (Purevdawa, Moon, Baigalmaa, Davaajav, Smith, and Vermund, 1997; Ramesh, Malla, Raju, Sehgal, Ganguly, Mahajan, and Dilawari, 1990). Bioterrorism may be favored because biological agents are relatively easy and inexpensive to obtain, can be easily disseminated, and can cause widespread fear and panic beyond the actual physical damage (Raut, 2004; Rehm, Mathers, Popova, Thavorncharoensap, Teerawattananon, and Patra, 2009; Rich and Perry, 2011). Military leaders, however, have learned that, as a military asset, bioterrorism has some important limitations (Rogers, Carolin, Vaught, and Compton, 2011; Ronohardjo and Rastiko, 1982; Sachs, 2001; Sachs and Malaney, 2002). First, it is difficult to use a bioweapon in a way that only affects the enemy and not friendly forces (Saleha, 1991; Sibert, Rigaud, Delavierre, and Labat, 2010; Skrepnek and Skrepnek, 2004; Sloane, 2009; Sockett, 1993). A biological weapon is useful to terrorists mainly as a method of creating mass panic and disruption to a state or a country (St George, 1986; Steben and Duarte-Franco, 2007; Stehr-Green and Schantz, 1987; Stuckler, 2008; Stuckler and Siegel, 2011). However, technologists such as Bill Joy have warned of the potential power which genetic engineering might place in the hands of future bio-terrorists (Suhrcke, Stuckler, Suk, Desai, Senek, McKee, and Rechel, 2011; Šumilo, Bormane, Asokliene, Vasilenko, Golovljova, Avsic-Zupanc, and Randolph, 2008). The use of agents that do not cause harm to humans, but disrupt the economy, have also been discussed (Tapia, 2003; Torgerson and Dowling, 2001; Torgerson, Carmona, and Bonifacino, 2000; Uddin Khan, Atanasova, Krueger, Ramirez, and Gray, 2013). One such pathogen is the foot-and-mouth disease virus, which is capable of causing widespread economic damage and public concern, while having almost no capacity to infect humans (Uusküla, Müürsepp, Kawai, Raag, Jürisson, and Pillsbury, 2013; Vanni, Karnon, Madan, White, Edmunds, Foss, and Legood, 2011). This chapter will close with a review of disease outbreaks that are due to changes in population profiles and genetics.

5.5. DISEASE OUTBREAKS DUE TO POPULATION PROFILES AND GENETICS

A genetic disorder is a health problem caused by one or more abnormalities in the genome (Yi-Xin and Manderson, 2005; Zadoks, 2008; Zhan, Li, Wang, Sun, Geng, Xiong, and de Hoog, 2015; Zhang, Song, Cai, and Zhou, 2008). It can be caused by a mutation in a single gene (monogenic) or multiple genes (polygenic) or by a chromosomal abnormality (Weycker, Edelsberg, Oster, and Tino, 2005; Wu, Perrings, Kinzig, Collins, Minteer, and Daszak, 2017; Yach, Stuckler, and Brownell, 2006). Although polygenic disorders are the most common, the term is mostly used when discussing disorders with a single genetic cause, either in a gene or chromosome (Casamassimo, Thikkurissy, Edelstein, and Maiorini, 2009; Castro, Wilson, and Bloom, 2017). The mutation responsible can occur spontaneously before embryonic development (a de novo mutation), or it can be inherited from two parents who are carriers of a faulty gene (autosomal recessive inheritance) or from a parent with the disorder or autosomal dominant inheritance (Narrod, Zinsstag, and Tiongco, 2012; Nascimento and de Oliveira, 2014; O'Brien, Lahue, Caro, and Davidson, 2007). Some disorders are caused by a mutation on the X chromosome and have X-linked inheritance. Very few disorders are inherited on the Y chromosome or mitochondrial DNA (Fenichel, 2013; Fenichel et al., 2011; Fogel, 1994). In Figure 5.5 we see that different chromosomes can be linked to specific diseases or genetic conditions (Daily, and Ehrlich, 1996; Deogaonkar, Hutubessy, Van Der Putten, Evers, and Jit, 2012; Dorn, 1992; Ducrotoy, Bertu, Ocholi, Gusi, Bryssinckx, Welburn, and Moriyon, 2014).

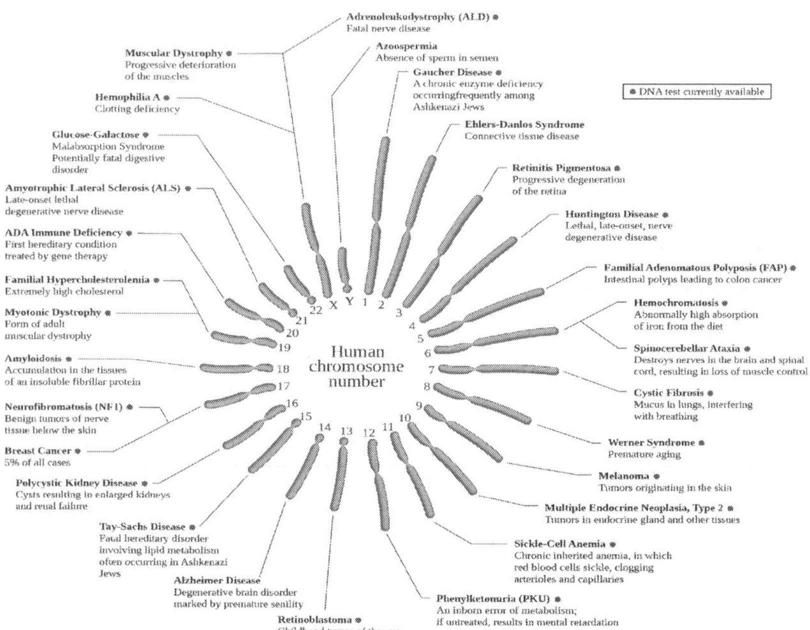

Figure 5.5. Human chromosomes that are linked to genetic diseases.

Source: Wikipedia.

There are well over 6,000 known genetic disorders and new genetic disorders are constantly being described in medical literature (Peckham, 2013; Perrings et al., 2002, 2014). Around 1 in 50 people are affected by a known single-gene disorder, while around 1 in 263 are affected by a chromosomal disorder (Saleha, 1991; Sibert, Rigaud, Delavierre, and Labat, 2010; Skrepnek and Skrepnek, 2004; Sloane, 2009; Sockett, 1993). Around

65% of people have some kind of health problem as a result of congenital genetic mutations (Tapia, 2003; Torgerson and Dowling, 2001; Torgerson, Carmona, and Bonifacino, 2000; Uddin Khan, Atanasova, Krueger, Ramirez, and Gray, 2013). Due to the significantly large number of genetic disorders, approximately 1 in 21 people are affected by a genetic disorder classified as "rare" (Borghol, Suderman, McArdle, Racine, Hallett, Pembrey, and Szyf, 2012; Brandes, 2008; Brown, Lipscomb, and Snyder, 2001). This is usually defined as affecting less than 1 in 2,000 people. Most genetic disorders are rare in themselves (Purevdawa, Moon, Baigalmaa, Davaajav, Smith, and Vermund, 1997; Ramesh, Malla, Raju, Sehgal, Ganguly, Mahajan, and Dilawari, 1990). Cancers are caused by genetic mutations but are generally omitted when referring to genetic disorders, since most are not hereditary (Bausch and Schwarz, 2014; Bausch et al., 2001; Benner, Carabin, Sánchez-Serrano, Budke, and Carmena, 2010). This is despite the fact that inherited predispositions and cancer syndromes exist (Rogers, Carolin, Vaught, and Compton, 2011; Ronohardjo and Rastiko, 1982; Sachs, 2001; Sachs and Malaney, 2002).

A single-gene disorder (or monogenic disorder) is the result of a single mutated gene (Oleś, Gudowska-Nowak, and Kleczkowski, 2012; Otte, Nugent, and McLeod, 2004; Ozawa, Portnoy, Getaneh, Clark, Knoll, Bishai, and Patwardhan, 2016). Single-gene disorders can be passed on to subsequent generations in several ways (Eaton and Groopman, 2013; Eckelman, Sherman, and MacNeill, 2018; Egger, 2011; Elbe, 2007; Ernst and Hay, 1994). Genomic imprinting and uniparental disomy, may nevertheless affect inheritance patterns (Moné, Ibikounlé, Massougbodji, and Mouahid, 2010; Morand, 2004; Moro, Budke, Schantz, Vasquez, Santivanez, and Villavicencio, 2011). The divisions between recessive and dominant types are not "hard and fast" (Foxman, 2002; Garner, Whan, Gard, and Phillips, 2001; Gayle and Hill, 2001; Gottstein, Pozio, and Nöckler, 2009). However, the divisions between autosomal and X-linked types are fairly set since the latter types are distinguished purely based on the chromosomal location of the gene (Markos and Abdela, 2016; Martin and Shepherd, 2009; McGuinness, McGlynn, Johnson, MacIntyre, Batty, Burns, and McGinty, 2012). For example, the common form of dwarfism, achondroplasia, is typically considered a dominant disorder (Hart and Halden, 2020; Häsler, Howe, and Stärk, 2011; Henschke, Kamper, and Maher, 2015; Hochberg, 1992). However, children with two genes for achondroplasia have a severe and usually lethal skeletal disorder, one that achondroplasics could be considered carriers for (Raut, 2004; Rehm,

Mathers, Popova, Thavorncharoensap, Teerawattananon, and Patra, 2009; Rich and Perry, 2011). Sickle-cell anemia is also considered a recessive condition, but heterozygous carriers have increased resistance to malaria in early childhood, which could be described as a related dominant condition (Howe, Häsler, and Stärk, 2013; Howe et al., 2012). When a couple where one partner or both are sufferers or carriers of a single-gene disorder wish to have a child, they can do so through in vitro fertilization, which enables preimplantation genetic diagnosis to occur to check whether the embryo has the genetic disorder (Arredondo and Zúñiga, 2006; Backer, van Roermund, Fischer, van Asseldonk, and Bergevoet, 2015; Bartsch, Hotez, Hertenstein, Diemert, Zapf, Bottazzi, and Lee, 2016).

Most congenital metabolic disorders known as inborn errors of metabolism result from single-gene defects (Bergevoet, Van Schaik, Veling, Backus, and Franken, 2009; Binder, 1988; Bolos, Bacarea, and Marusteri, 2011). Many such single-gene defects can decrease the fitness of affected people and are therefore present in the population in lower frequencies compared to what would be expected based on simple probabilistic calculations (Suhrcke, Stuckler, Suk, Desai, Senek, McKee, and Rechel, 2011; Šumilo, Bormane, Asokliene, Vasilenko, Golovljova, Avsic-Zupanc, and Randolph, 2008). Only one mutated copy of the gene will be necessary for a person to be affected by an autosomal dominant disorder (Poundstone, Strathdee, and Celentano, 2004; Pritchett, Thilmany, and Johnson, 2005; Pugliatti, Beghi, Forsgren, Ekman, and Sobocki, 2007). Each affected person usually has one affected parent (Armelagos, Brown, and Turner, 2005; Arokiasamy and Krishnan, 1994; Arora, 2001, 2005; Arredondo and Zúñiga, 2004). The chance a child will inherit the mutated gene is 50% (Krieger, 2001a, b; Lemma, 1969; Liu, Maniadakis, Gray, and Rayner, 2002; López, Torné, Franco, San-Martin, Viayna, Barrull, and Perulero, 2018). Autosomal dominant conditions sometimes have reduced penetrance, which means although only one mutated copy is needed, not all individuals who inherit that mutation go on to develop the disease (Amuna and Zotor, 2008; Aral, Holmes, Padian, and Cates, 1996; Arbabi, Nezami, Hooshyar, and Delavari, 2018). Examples of this type of disorder are Huntington's disease, neurofibromatosis type 1, neurofibromatosis type 2, Marfan syndrome, hereditary nonpolyposis colorectal cancer, hereditary multiple exostoses (which is a highly penetrant autosomal dominant disorder), tuberous sclerosis, Von Willebrand disease, and acute intermittent porphyria (St George, 1986; Steben and Duarte-Franco, 2007; Stehr-Green and Schantz, 1987; Stuckler, 2008; Stuckler and Siegel, 2011). Birth defects are also called congenital anomalies (Acemoglu and Johnson, 2007; Adda, 2016; Alloul, Sauriol, Kennedy, Laurier, Tessier, Novosel, and Contandriopoulos, 1998).

Two copies of the gene must be mutated for a person to be affected by an autosomal recessive disorder (Uusküla, Müürsepp, Kawai, Raag, Jürisson, and Pillsbury, 2013; Vanni, Karnon, Madan, White, Edmunds, Foss, and Legood, 2011). An affected person usually has unaffected parents who each carry a single copy of the mutated gene and are referred to as genetic carriers (Perry and Randolph, 1999; Philipson, 2000; Philipson and Posner, 1996; Pongchaiyakul, Songpattanasilp, and Taechakraichana, 2008). Each parent with a defective gene normally do not have symptoms (Weycker, Edelsberg, Oster, and Tino, 2005; Wu, Perrings, Kinzig, Collins, Minteer, and Daszak, 2017; Yach, Stuckler, and Brownell, 2006). Two unaffected people who each carry one copy of the mutated gene have a 25% risk with each pregnancy of having a child affected by the disorder (Chen, Li, Hsieh, Chang, Lee, Lee, and Ko, 2012; Conover, Pitt, Kessler, DuBow, and Sanborn, 1995; Crump, Murdoch, and Baker, 2001). Examples of this type of disorder are albinism, medium-chain Acyl-CoA dehydrogenase deficiency, cystic fibrosis, sickle cell disease, Tay-Sachs disease, Niemann-Pick disease, spinal muscular atrophy, and Roberts syndrome (Kim and Goldie, 2008; Klein, Laxminarayan, Smith, and Gilligan, 2007; Klepac, Laxminarayan, and Grenfell, 2011). Certain other phenotypes, such as wet versus dry earwax, are also determined in an autosomal recessive fashion (Abegunde and Stanciole, 2008; Abramowitz, Lacau Saint Guily, Moyal-Barracco, Bergeron, Borne, Dahlab, and Bénard, 2018). Some autosomal recessive disorders are common because, in the past, carrying one of the faulty genes led to a slight protection against an infectious disease or toxin such as tuberculosis or malaria (Jenkins, Baingana, Ahmad, McDaid, and Atun, 2011; Johnson, Alvarez-Pasquin, Bijl, Franco, Gaillat, Clara, and Weinke, 2015). Such disorders include cystic fibrosis, sickle cell disease, phenylketonuria, and thalassemia (Pal, Kerorsa, Marami, and Kandi, 2020; Paterson, Otte, Slingenbergh, Wint, and Rogers, 2000; Pearce and Merletti, 2006).

X-linked dominant disorders are caused by mutations in genes on the X chromosome (Yi-Xin and Manderson, 2005; Zadoks, 2008; Zhan, Li, Wang, Sun, Geng, Xiong, and de Hoog, 2015; Zhang, Song, Cai, and Zhou, 2008). Only a few disorders have this inheritance pattern, with a prime example being X-linked hypophosphatemic rickets (Bwire, Munier, Ouedraogo, Heyerdahl, Komakech, Kagirita, and Makumbi, 2017; Canali, Aragrande, Angheben, Capelli, Drigo, Gobbi, and Cassini, 2020). Males and females are both affected in these disorders, with males typically being more severely affected than females (Buckley, 1984; Budke, Jiamin, Qian, and Torgerson, 2005; Bundy, Arámbulo III, and Grey, 1983; Buzby and Roberts, 2009). Some X-linked dominant conditions, such as Rett syndrome, incontinentia pigmenti type 2, and Aicardi syndrome, are usually fatal in males either in utero or shortly after birth, and are therefore predominantly seen in females (Espinoza, Terashima, Herrera-Velit, and Marcos, 2010; Ezzati, Vander Hoorn, Lawes, Leach, James, Lopez, and Murray, 2005). Exceptions to this finding are extremely rare cases in which boys with Klinefelter syndrome (44+xxy) also inherit an X-linked dominant condition and exhibit symptoms more similar to those of a female in terms of disease severity (Bonds, Keenan, Rohani, and Sachs, 2010; Boni, Galvani, Wickelgren, and Malani, 2013; Bonovas and Nikolopoulos, 2012). The chance of passing on an X-linked dominant disorder differs between men and women (Ozmen, Kurşun, and Ozcelik, 2005; Paarlberg, Hillberg, Lee, and Mathews, 2008; Paisley, Vraa-Andersen, Dybkjaer, Møller, Christensen, Mousing, and Agger, 1993). The sons of a man with an X-linked dominant disorder will all be unaffected (since they receive their father's Y chromosome), but his daughters will all inherit the condition (Casamassimo, Thikkurissy, Edelstein, and Maiorini, 2009; Castro, Wilson, and Bloom, 2017). A woman with an X-linked dominant disorder has a 50% chance of having an affected fetus with each pregnancy, although in cases such as incontinentia pigmenti, only female offspring are generally viable (Poundstone, Strathdee, and Celentano, 2004; Pritchett, Thilmany, and Johnson, 2005; Pugliatti, Beghi, Forsgren, Ekman, and Sobocki, 2007).

CHAPTER 5 SUMMARY

Disease can emanate in different modalities which are directly linked to their causes. These differentiated modalities allow for the classification of disease epidemicsDisease epidemics as being common source, propagated, contagious, non-contagious, artificial, and genetic. The next two chapters summarizes the modes of transmission and their implications for the management of the epidemics.

Chapter

6

Modes of Transmission for Disease epidemics Part 1

CONTENTS

The mode of transmission for a disease epidemic will impact on all the public safety measures that are taken in response. This chapter is the first of two penultimate chapters considering this particular aspect of disease epidemiology and management. The key modalities that will be examined in this chapter include diseases that are transmitted through air, arthropods, biological methods, contact, and Cyclopropagative means. By the end of this chapter, the reader should have a general idea of how these transmission modalities determine the impact of a disease epidemic.

6.1. AIRBORNE TRANSMISSION OF DISEASE EPIDEMIC

An airborne transmission is disease transmission through small particulates that can be transmitted through the air over time and distance (St George, 1986; Steben and Duarte-Franco, 2007; Stehr-Green and Schantz, 1987; Stuckler, 2008; Stuckler and Siegel, 2011). Diseases capable of airborne transmission include many of considerable importance both in human and veterinary medicine (Kim and Goldie, 2008; Klein, Laxminarayan, Smith, and Gilligan, 2007; Klepac, Laxminarayan, and Grenfell, 2011). The relevant pathogens may be viruses, bacteria, or fungi, and they may be spread through breathing, talking, coughing, sneezing, raising of dust, spraying of liquids, toilet flushing or any activities which generate aerosol particles or droplets (Bonds, Keenan, Rohani, and Sachs, 2010; Boni, Galvani, Wickelgren, and Malani, 2013; Bonovas and Nikolopoulos, 2012). Human airborne diseases do not include conditions caused by air pollution such as volatile organic compounds, gases, and any airborne particles (Oleś, Gudowska-Nowak, and Kleczkowski, 2012; Otte, Nugent, and McLeod, 2004; Ozawa, Portnoy, Getaneh, Clark, Knoll, Bishai, and Patwardhan, 2016). In Figure 6.1, we see an illustration of how airborne diseases are transmitted.

Airborne transmission is distinct from transmission by respiratory droplets (Armelagos, Brown, and Turner, 2005; Arokiasamy and Krishnan, 1994; Arora, 2001, 2005; Arredondo and Zúñiga, 2004). Respiratory droplets are large enough to fall to the ground rapidly after being produced (usually greater than 5 μm), although this arbitrary cutoff has never been demonstrated experimentally or supported theoretically, as opposed to the smaller particles that carry airborne pathogens (Bwire, Munier, Ouedraogo, Heyerdahl, Komakech, Kagirita, and Makumbi, 2017; Canali, Aragrande, Angheben, Capelli, Drigo, Gobbi, and Cassini, 2020).

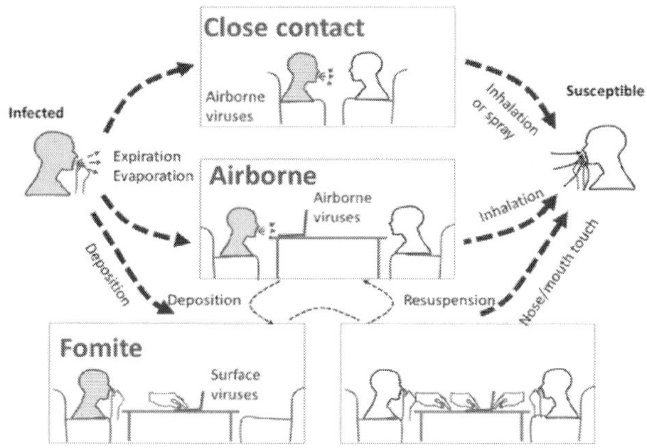

Figure 6.1. Transmission of airborne diseases.

Source: BMC Infectious Diseases.

Moreover, while respiratory droplets consist mostly of water; airborne particles are relatively dry (Borghol, Suderman, McArdle, Racine, Hallett, Pembrey, and Szyf, 2012; Brandes, 2008; Brown, Lipscomb, and Snyder, 2001). This damages many pathogens so that their ability to transmit infection is lessened or eliminated (Peckham, 2013; Perrings et al., 2002, 2014). Thus the number of pathogens that can be transmitted through an airborne route is limited (Amuna and Zotor, 2008; Aral, Holmes, Padian, and Cates, 1996; Arbabi, Nezami, Hooshyar, and Delavari, 2018). Airborne diseases include any that are caused via transmission through the air (Acemoglu and Johnson, 2007; Adda, 2016; Alloul, Sauriol, Kennedy, Laurier, Tessier, Novosel, and Contandriopoulos, 1998).

Many airborne diseases are of great medical importance (Eaton and Groopman, 2013; Eckelman, Sherman, and MacNeill, 2018; Egger, 2011; Elbe, 2007; Ernst and Hay, 1994). The pathogens transmitted may be any kind of microbe, and they may be spread in aerosols, dust or liquids (Espinoza, Terashima, Herrera-Velit, and Marcos, 2010; Ezzati, Vander Hoorn, Lawes, Leach, James, Lopez, and Murray, 2005). The aerosols might be generated from sources of infection such as the bodily secretions of an infected animal or person, or biological wastes such as accumulate in lofts, caves, garbage, and the like (Markos and Abdela, 2016; Martin and Shepherd, 2009; McGuinness, McGlynn, Johnson, MacIntyre, Batty, Burns, and McGinty, 2012). Such infected aerosols may stay suspended in air currents long enough to travel for considerable distances (Suhrcke, Stuckler,

Suk, Desai, Senek, McKee, and Rechel, 2011; Šumilo, Bormane, Asokliene, Vasilenko, Golovljova, Avsic-Zupanc, and Randolph, 2008).

Airborne pathogens or allergens often cause inflammation in the nose, throat, sinuses, and the lungs (Bergevoet, Van Schaik, Veling, Backus, and Franken, 2009; Binder, 1988; Bolos, Bacarea, and Marusteri, 2011). This is caused by the inhalation of these pathogens that affect a person's respiratory system or even the rest of the body (Tapia, 2003; Torgerson and Dowling, 2001; Torgerson, Carmona, and Bonifacino, 2000; Uddin Khan, Atanasova, Krueger, Ramirez, and Gray, 2013). Sinus congestion, coughing, and sore throats are examples of inflammation of the upper respiratory airway due to these airborne agents (Moné, Ibikounlé, Massougbodji, and Mouahid, 2010; Morand, 2004; Moro, Budke, Schantz, Vasquez, Santivanez, and Villavicencio, 2011). Air pollution plays a significant role in airborne diseases which is linked to asthma (Uusküla, Müürsepp, Kawai, Raag, Jürisson, and Pillsbury, 2013; Vanni, Karnon, Madan, White, Edmunds, Foss, and Legood, 2011). Pollutants are said to influence lung function by increasing airway inflammation (Raut, 2004; Rehm, Mathers, Popova, Thavorncharoensap, Teerawattananon, and Patra, 2009; Rich and Perry, 2011). Many common infections can spread by airborne transmission at least in some cases, including but not limited to: measles morbillivirus, chickenpox virus; Mycobacterium tuberculosis, influenza virus, enterovirus, norovirus, and less commonly coronavirus, adenovirus, and possibly respiratory syncytial virus (Foxman, 2002; Garner, Whan, Gard, and Phillips, 2001; Gayle and Hill, 2001; Gottstein, Pozio, and Nöckler, 2009). Because the drying process often damages the pathogens, the number of diseases that can be spread through an airborne route is limited (Howe, Häsler, and Stärk, 2013; Howe et al., 2012).

Airborne diseases can also affect non-humans (Weycker, Edelsberg, Oster, and Tino, 2005; Wu, Perrings, Kinzig, Collins, Minteer, and Daszak, 2017; Yach, Stuckler, and Brownell, 2006). For example, New castle disease is an avian disease that affects many types of domestic poultry worldwide which is transmitted via airborne contamination (Daily, and Ehrlich, 1996; Deogaonkar, Hutubessy, Van Der Putten, Evers, and Jit, 2012; Dorn, 1992; Ducrotoy, Bertu, Ocholi, Gusi, Bryssinckx, Welburn, and Moriyon, 2014). Often, airborne pathogens or allergens cause inflammation in the nose, throat, sinuses, and the upper airway lungs (Chen, Li, Hsieh, Chang, Lee, Lee, and Ko, 2012; Conover, Pitt, Kessler, DuBow, and Sanborn, 1995; Crump, Murdoch, and Baker, 2001);. Upper airway inflammation causes coughing congestion, and sore throat (Arredondo and Zúñiga, 2006; Backer, van Roermund, Fischer, van Asseldonk, and Bergevoet, 2015; Bartsch, Hotez, Hertenstein, Diemert, Zapf, Bottazzi, and Lee, 2016). This is caused by the inhalation of these pathogens that affect a person's respiratory system or even the rest of the body (Rogers, Carolin, Vaught, and Compton, 2011; Ronohardjo and Rastiko, 1982; Sachs, 2001; Sachs and Malaney, 2002). Sinus congestion, coughing, and sore throats are examples of inflammation of the upper respiratory airway due to these airborne agents (Yi-Xin and Manderson, 2005; Zadoks, 2008; Zhan, Li, Wang, Sun, Geng, Xiong, and de Hoog, 2015; Zhang, Song, Cai, and Zhou, 2008). The next section considers diseases that occur through arthropod transmission.

6.2. ARTHROPOD TRANSMISSION OF DISEASE EPIDEMICS

Anthroponosis refers to pathogens sourced from humans and can include human to non-human animal transmission but also human to human transmission (Perry and Randolph, 1999; Philipson, 2000; Philipson and Posner, 1996; Pongchaiyakul, Songpattanasilp, and Taechakraichana, 2008). The term zoonosis technically refers to disease transferred between any animal and another animal, human or non-human, without discretion, and also been defined as disease transmitted from animals to humans and vice versa (Abegunde and Stanciole, 2008; Abramowitz, Lacau Saint Guily, Moyal-Barracco, Bergeron, Borne, Dahlab, and Bénard, 2018). Yet because of human-centered medical biases, zoonosis tends to be used in the same manner as anthropozoonosis, which specifically refers to pathogens reservoired in non-human animals that are transmissible to humans (Fenichel, 2013; Fenichel et al., 2011; Fogel, 1994). Additional confusion due to frequency of scientists using "anthropozoonosis" and "zooanthroponosis" interchangeably was resolved during 1967; Joint Food and Agriculture and World Health Organization (WHO) committee meeting that recommended the use of "zoonosis" to describe the bidirectional interchange of infectious pathogens between animals and humans (Saleha, 1991; Sibert, Rigaud, Delavierre, and Labat, 2010; Skrepnek and Skrepnek, 2004; Sloane, 2009; Sockett, 1993). Figure 6.2 highlights how an arthropod-borne disease can be transmitted from one human being to another.

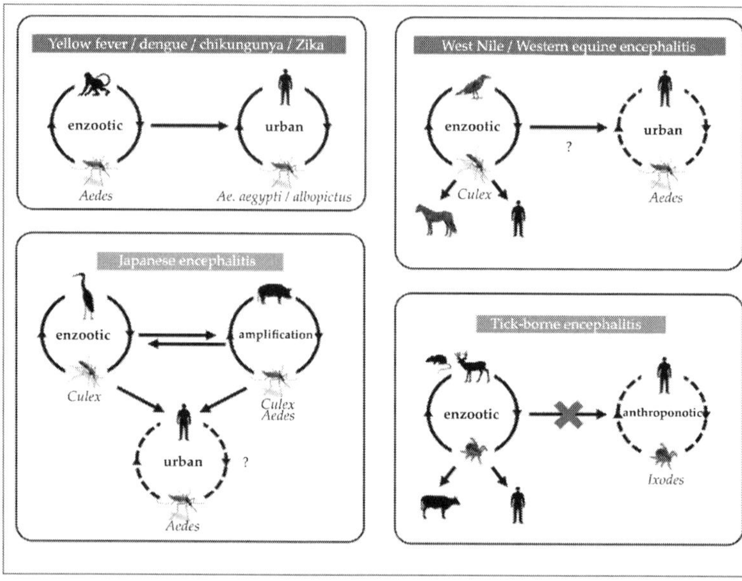

Figure 6.2. Human to human transmission of arthropod-borne pathogens.

Source: Science Direct.

Furthermore, because humans are rarely in direct contact with wild animals and introduce pathogens through "soft contact," the term "sapronotic agents" must be introduced (Bausch and Schwarz, 2014; Bausch et al., 2001; Benner, Carabin, Sánchez-Serrano, Budke, and Carmena, 2010). Sapronoses refers to human diseases that harbor the capacity to grow and replicate (not just survive or contaminate) in abiotic environments such as soil, water, decaying plants, animal corpses, excreta, and other substrate (Hart and Halden, 2020; Häsler, Howe, and Stärk, 2011; Henschke, Kamper, and Maher, 2015; Hochberg, 1992). Additionally, sapro-zoonoses can be characterized as having both a live host and a non-animal developmental site of organic matter, soil, or plants (Ozmen, Kurşun, and Ozcelik, 2005; Paarlberg, Hillberg, Lee, and Mathews, 2008; Paisley, Vraa-Andersen, Dybkjaer, Møller, Christensen, Mousing, and Agger, 1993). It must be noted that obligate intracellular parasites that cannot replicate outside of cells and are entirely reproductively reliant on entering the cell to use intracellular resources such as viruses, rickettsiae, chlamydiae, and Cryptosporidium parvum cannot be sapronotic agents (Buckley, 1984; Budke, Jiamin, Qian, and Torgerson, 2005; Bundy, Arámbulo III, and Grey, 1983; Buzby and Roberts, 2009). Categorizing of disease into epidemiologic classes by the infection's supposed source or the direction of transmission raises a number of contradictions that could be resolved by the use of cyclical models as demonstrated by a number of scenarios.

First is the distinction between Zoonosis, reverse zoonosis, and Anthroponosis (Narrod, Zinsstag, and Tiongco, 2012; Nascimento and de Oliveira, 2014; O'Brien, Lahue, Caro, and Davidson, 2007). In the case of diseases transferred from arthropod vectors (such as urban yellow fever, dengue, epidemic typhus, tick-borne relapsing fever, Zika fever, and malaria), the differentiation between terms becomes even less clear (Pal, Kerorsa, Marami, and Kandi, 2020; Paterson, Otte, Slingenbergh, Wint, and Rogers, 2000; Pearce and Merletti, 2006). For example, a human infected with malaria is bitten by a mosquito that is subsequently infected as well. This is a case of reverse zoonosis (human to animal). However, the newly infected mosquito then infects another human. This could be a case of zoonosis (animal to human) if the mosquito is considered the original source, or Anthroponosis (human to human) if the human is considered the original source. If this infected mosquito instead infected a non-human primate, it could be considered a case of reverse zoonosis or zooanthroponosis (human to animal) if the human is considered the primary source. It could also be simply zoonosis (animal to animal) if the mosquito is considered the primary source.

The second scenario is the distinction between Zoonosis vs anthroponosis (Krieger, 2001a, b; Lemma, 1969; Liu, Maniadakis, Gray, and Rayner, 2002; López, Torné, Franco, San-Martin, Viayna, Barrull, and Perulero, 2018). HIV originating in simians (crossover due to humans consuming wild chimpanzee bushmeat) and influenza A viruses originating in avians (crossover due to an antigenic shift) could have initially been considered a zoonotic transference as the infections first came from vertebrate animals (Jenkins, Baingana, Ahmad, McDaid, and Atun, 2011; Johnson, Alvarez-Pasquin, Bijl, Franco, Gaillat, Clara, and Weinke, 2015). However, it could also currently be regarded as an anthroponosis because of its potential to transfer between human to human (Purevdawa, Moon, Baigalmaa, Davaajav, Smith, and Vermund, 1997; Ramesh, Malla, Raju, Sehgal, Ganguly, Mahajan, and Dilawari, 1990). An alternative example is the scenario of distinguishing between Sapronosis and sapro-zoonosis (Jenkins, Baingana, Ahmad, McDaid, and Atun, 2011; Johnson, Alvarez-Pasquin, Bijl, Franco, Gaillat, Clara, and Weinke, 2015). Typical examples of sapronotic agents are fungal such as coccidioidomycosis, histoplasmosis, aspergillosis, cryptococcosis, *Microsporum gypseum* (Krieger, 2001a, b; Lemma, 1969; Liu, Maniadakis,

Gray, and Rayner, 2002; López, Torné, Franco, San-Martin, Viayna, Barrull, and Perulero, 2018). Some can be bacterial from the sporulating clostridium and bacillus to *Rhodococcus equi*, *Burkholderia pseudomallei*, Listeria, Erysipelothrix, *Yersinia pseudotuberculosis*, legionellosis, Pontiac fever, and nontuberculous mycobacteriosis (Narrod, Zinsstag, and Tiongco, 2012; Nascimento and de Oliveira, 2014; O'Brien, Lahue, Caro, and Davidson, 2007). Other sapronotic agents are amebic as in primary amebic meningoencephalitis (Pal, Kerorsa, Marami, and Kandi, 2020; Paterson, Otte, Slingenbergh, Wint, and Rogers, 2000; Pearce and Merletti, 2006). Yet again, difficulties in classification arise in the case of sporulating bacteria whose infectious spores are only produced after a significant period of inactive vegetative growth within an abiotic environment (Buckley, 1984; Budke, Jiamin, Qian, and Torgerson, 2005; Bundy, Arámbulo III, and Grey, 1983; Buzby and Roberts, 2009). However, this is still considered a case of sapronoses (Ozmen, Kurşun, and Ozcelik, 2005; Paarlberg, Hillberg, Lee, and Mathews, 2008; Paisley, Vraa-Andersen, Dybkjaer, Møller, Christensen, Mousing, and Agger, 1993). Nevertheless, cases of zoo-sapronoses involving Listeria, Erysipelothrix, *Yersinia pseudotuberculosis*, *Burkholderia pseudomallei*, and *Rhodococcus equi* can be transferred by an animal or an abiotic substrate (Hart and Halden, 2020; Häsler, Howe, and Stärk, 2011; Henschke, Kamper, and Maher, 2015; Hochberg, 1992). The difference is that they usually occur via a fecal-oral route between humans and other animals (Bausch and Schwarz, 2014; Bausch et al., 2001; Benner, Carabin, Sánchez-Serrano, Budke, and Carmena, 2010).

There are certain cases which are linked to specific modes of transmission and via arthropod vectors (Saleha, 1991; Sibert, Rigaud, Delavierre, and Labat, 2010; Skrepnek and Skrepnek, 2004; Sloane, 2009; Sockett, 1993). A case in point is the malaria parasite whose life cycle is played out in hosts (Fenichel, 2013; Fenichel et al., 2011; Fogel, 1994). Malaria involves the cyclical infection of animals (human and non-human) and mosquitoes from the genus Anopheles with a number of Plasmodium species (Abegunde and Stanciole, 2008; Abramowitz, Lacau Saint Guily, Moyal-Barracco, Bergeron, Borne, Dahlab, and Bénard, 2018). The Plasmodium parasite is transferred to the mosquito as it feeds on the blood of the infected animal whereupon it begins a sporogenic cycle in the gut of the mosquito that will infect another animal at the next blood meal (Perry and Randolph, 1999; Philipson, 2000; Philipson and Posner, 1996; Pongchaiyakul, Songpattanasilp, and Taechakraichana, 2008). There does not seem to be any deleterious effects to the mosquito as a result of the parasitic infection (Yi-Xin and Manderson,

2005; Zadoks, 2008; Zhan, Li, Wang, Sun, Geng, Xiong, and de Hoog, 2015; Zhang, Song, Cai, and Zhou, 2008).

The *Plasmodium brasilianum* parasite normally found in primates is morphologically similar to the malarial inducing *Plasmodium malariae* that is more commonly found in humans and it is contested as to whether the two are actually different species (Rogers, Carolin, Vaught, and Compton, 2011; Ronohardjo and Rastiko, 1982; Sachs, 2001; Sachs and Malaney, 2002). Nevertheless, 12 reports of malaria in the remotely located indigenous Yanomami communities of the Venezuelan Amazon arose where it was surprisingly found to be caused by a strain of *P. brasilianum* with 100% identical to sequences found in Alouatta seniculus monkeys (Arredondo and Zúñiga, 2006; Backer, van Roermund, Fischer, van Asseldonk, and Bergevoet, 2015; Bartsch, Hotez, Hertenstein, Diemert, Zapf, Bottazzi, and Lee, 2016). This suggests a definite zoonosis and high possibility of spillback back into non-human primate bands as reverse zoonoses (Chen, Li, Hsieh, Chang, Lee, Lee, and Ko, 2012; Conover, Pitt, Kessler, DuBow, and Sanborn, 1995; Crump, Murdoch, and Baker, 2001).

Trypanosoma brucei gambiense (*T. b. gambiense*) is a species of African trypanosomes which are protozoan hemoflagellates responsible for trypanosomiasis (more commonly known as African sleeping sickness) in humans and other animals (Daily, and Ehrlich, 1996; Deogaonkar, Hutubessy, Van Der Putten, Evers, and Jit, 2012; Dorn, 1992; Ducrotoy, Bertu, Ocholi, Gusi, Bryssinckx, Welburn, and Moriyon, 2014). The protozoa are transferred via Tsetse flies where they multiply and can be transferred to yet another animal host during the fly's blood meal feeding (Weycker, Edelsberg, Oster, and Tino, 2005; Wu, Perrings, Kinzig, Collins, Minteer, and Daszak, 2017; Yach, Stuckler, and Brownell, 2006). Outbreaks of sleeping sickness in certain human communities have been eliminated but only temporarily as constant re-introduction from unknown sources statistically suggests the presence of a non-human reservoir where spillback of the pathogen is maintained in a sylvatic cycle and re-introduced into the urban cycle (Howe, Häsler, and Stärk, 2013; Howe et al., 2012). The presence of *T. b. gambiense* has been found separately in humans and livestock (Foxman, 2002; Garner, Whan, Gard, and Phillips, 2001; Gayle and Hill, 2001; Gottstein, Pozio, and Nöckler, 2009). This spurred a molecular study comparing serum reactivity of pigs, goats, and cows to human serum where notable similarities in all samples but especially in pig samples (Raut, 2004; Rehm, Mathers, Popova, Thavorncharoensap, Teerawattananon, and Patra, 2009; Rich and Perry, 2011). Combined, these findings implicate a reverse zoonotic human to animal transmission (Uusküla, Müürsepp, Kawai, Raag, Jürisson, and Pillsbury, 2013; Vanni, Karnon, Madan, White, Edmunds, Foss, and Legood, 2011). The next section summarizes the biological transmission of disease epidemicsDisease epidemics.

6.3. CONTACT TRANSMISSION OF DISEASE EPIDEMICS

Contact transmission is an important consideration when managing disease epidemicsDisease epidemics (Moné, Ibikounlé, Massougbodji, and Mouahid, 2010; Morand, 2004; Moro, Budke, Schantz, Vasquez, Santivanez, and Villavicencio, 2011). Transmission of an infection requires three conditions (Tapia, 2003; Torgerson and Dowling, 2001; Torgerson, Carmona, and Bonifacino, 2000; Uddin Khan, Atanasova, Krueger, Ramirez, and Gray, 2013). First, there must be an infectious individual. Secondly, there must be a susceptible individual (Bergevoet, Van Schaik, Veling, Backus, and Franken, 2009; Binder, 1988; Bolos, Bacarea, and Marusteri, 2011). Thirdly there must be an effective contact between them (Suhrcke, Stuckler, Suk, Desai, Senek, McKee, and Rechel, 2011; Šumilo, Bormane, Asokliene, Vasilenko, Golovljova, Avsic-Zupanc, and Randolph, 2008). An effective contact is defined as any kind of contact between two individuals such that, if one individual is infectious and the other susceptible, then the first individual infects the second (Markos and Abdela, 2016; Martin and Shepherd, 2009; McGuinness, McGlynn, Johnson, MacIntyre, Batty, Burns, and McGinty, 2012). Whether or not a particular kind of contact will be effective depends on the infectious agent and its route of transmission (Espinoza, Terashima, Herrera-Velit, and Marcos, 2010; Ezzati, Vander Hoorn, Lawes, Leach, James, Lopez, and Murray, 2005). The effective contact rate (denoted β) in a given population for a given infectious disease is measured in effective contacts per unit time (Eaton and Groopman, 2013; Eckelman, Sherman, and MacNeill, 2018; Egger, 2011; Elbe, 2007; Ernst and Hay, 1994). Figure 6.3 is an illustration of the direct and indirect disease transmission modalities.

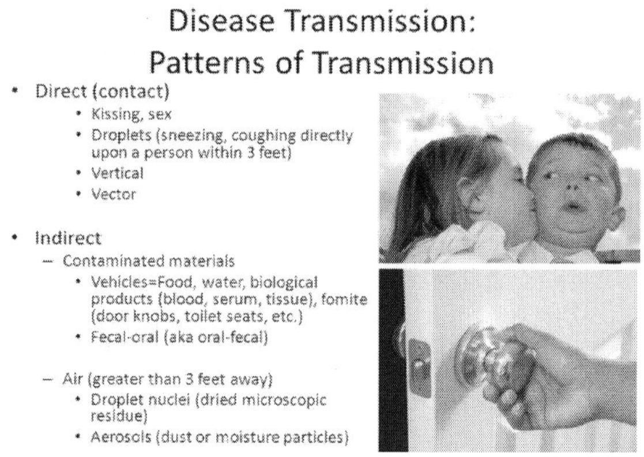

Figure 6.3. Direct and indirect disease transmission modalities.

Source: Slide Player.

This may be expressed as the total contact rate (the total number of contacts, effective or not, per unit time, denoted γ, multiplied by the risk of infection, given contact between an infectious and a susceptible individual (Acemoglu and Johnson, 2007; Adda, 2016; Alloul, Sauriol, Kennedy, Laurier, Tessier, Novosel, and Contandriopoulos, 1998). This risk is called the transmission risk and is denoted p. The total contact rate γ will generally be greater than the effective contact rate β, since not all contacts result in infection. That is to say, p is almost always less than 1, and it can never be greater than 1, since it is effectively the probability of transmission occurring. This relation formalizes the fact that the effective contact rate depends not only on the social patterns of contact in a particular society (γ) but also on the specific types of contact and the pathology of the infectious organism (p). For example, it has been shown that a concurrent sexually transmitted infection can substantially increase the probability (p) of infecting a susceptible with HIV (Amuna and Zotor, 2008; Aral, Holmes, Padian, and Cates, 1996; Arbabi, Nezami, Hooshyar, and Delavari, 2018). Therefore, one way to reduce the value of p (and hence lower HIV transmission rates) might be to treat other sexually transmitted infections (Peckham, 2013; Perrings et al., 2002, 2014).

There are a number of difficulties in using this relation (Borghol, Suderman, McArdle, Racine, Hallett, Pembrey, and Szyf, 2012; Brandes, 2008; Brown, Lipscomb, and Snyder, 2001). The first is that it is very difficult to measure contact rates because they vary widely between individuals and groups, and within the same group at different times (Bwire, Munier, Ouedraogo, Heyerdahl, Komakech, Kagirita, and Makumbi, 2017; Canali, Aragrande, Angheben, Capelli, Drigo, Gobbi, and Cassini, 2020). For sexually transmitted infections, large scale studies of sexual behavior have been set up to estimate the contact rate (Armelagos, Brown, and Turner, 2005; Arokiasamy and Krishnan, 1994; Arora, 2001, 2005; Arredondo and Zúñiga, 2004). In developed countries for serious diseases such as AIDS or tuberculosis, contact tracing is often carried out when a patient is diagnosed (Oleś, Gudowska-Nowak, and Kleczkowski, 2012; Otte, Nugent, and McLeod, 2004; Ozawa, Portnoy, Getaneh, Clark, Knoll, Bishai, and Patwardhan, 2016). Here, the patient and medical authorities try to inform every possible contact the patient may have made since infection (Bonds, Keenan, Rohani, and Sachs, 2010; Boni, Galvani, Wickelgren, and Malani, 2013; Bonovas and Nikolopoulos, 2012). This, however, is not so much a research tool and more to alert the contacts to the possibility that they may be infected and so can seek medical treatment and avoiding passing on the disease if they have contracted it (Kim and Goldie, 2008; Klein, Laxminarayan, Smith, and Gilligan, 2007; Klepac, Laxminarayan, and Grenfell, 2011). A second consideration is that it is generally thought unethical to carry out direct experiments to establish per-contact infection risks as this would require the deliberate exposure of individuals to infectious agents (St George, 1986; Steben and Duarte-Franco, 2007; Stehr-Green and Schantz, 1987; Stuckler, 2008; Stuckler and Siegel, 2011). The Common Cold Unit that researched cold transmission in the UK between 1946 and 1989 was a notable exception (Poundstone, Strathdee, and Celentano, 2004; Pritchett, Thilmany, and Johnson, 2005; Pugliatti, Beghi, Forsgren, Ekman, and Sobocki, 2007). It is also possible to estimate the transmission risk in certain circumstances where exposures to infection have been documented (Casamassimo, Thikkurissy, Edelstein, and Maiorini, 2009; Castro, Wilson, and Bloom, 2017). For example, the rate of infection among nurses who have accidentally pricked their fingers with a needle that had previously been used with contaminated blood (Yi-Xin and Manderson, 2005; Zadoks, 2008; Zhan, Li, Wang, Sun, Geng, Xiong, and de Hoog, 2015; Zhang, Song, Cai, and Zhou, 2008). A more direct assessment of transmission risks can be provided by a contact study, which is often carried out because of an outbreak (Weycker, Edelsberg, Oster, and Tino, 2005; Wu, Perrings, Kinzig, Collins, Minteer, and Daszak, 2017; Yach, Stuckler, and Brownell, 2006). A notable example is a study was carried out during the SARS outbreak of 2002–2003.

CHAPTER 6 SUMMARY

This chapter has considered a range of transmission modalities for epidemics. These include diseases that are transmitted by air, arthropods, and through contact. The next chapter continues with this theme by examining other modalities of disease transmission.

Chapter 7

Modes of Transmission for Disease Epidemics Part 2

CONTENTS

As a continuation of the disease transmission themes, we will examine a number of pathways and their implications for public health. Some of these include developmental issues, fecal-oral routes, horizontal transmission, propagative transmission, and vertical transmission. By the end of this chapter, the reader will have a broad view of transmission modalities and how they impact on responses to disease epidemics.

7.1. FECAL-ORAL TRANSMISSION OF DISEASE EPIDEMICS

The fecal-oral route (also called the oral-fecal route or orofecal route) describes a particular route of transmission of a disease wherein pathogens in fecal particles pass from one person to the mouth of another person (Uusküla, Müürsepp, Kawai, Raag, Jürisson, and Pillsbury, 2013; Vanni, Karnon, Madan, White, Edmunds, Foss, and Legood, 2011). Main causes of fecal-oral disease transmission include lack of adequate sanitation (leading to open defecation), and poor hygiene practices (Tapia, 2003; Torgerson and Dowling, 2001; Torgerson, Carmona, and Bonifacino, 2000; Uddin Khan, Atanasova, Krueger, Ramirez, and Gray, 2013). If soil or water bodies are polluted with fecal material, humans can be infected with waterborne diseases or soil-transmitted diseases (Suhrcke, Stuckler, Suk, Desai, Senek, McKee, and Rechel, 2011; Šumilo, Bormane, Asokliene, Vasilenko, Golovljova, Avsic-Zupanc, and Randolph, 2008). Fecal contamination of food is another form of fecal-oral transmission (St George, 1986; Steben and Duarte-Franco, 2007; Stehr-Green and Schantz, 1987; Stuckler, 2008; Stuckler and Siegel, 2011). Washing hands properly after changing a baby's diaper or after performing anal hygiene can prevent foodborne illness from spreading (Saleha, 1991; Sibert, Rigaud, Delavierre, and Labat, 2010; Skrepnek and Skrepnek, 2004; Sloane, 2009; Sockett, 1993). Figure 7.1 is a demonstration of the main modalities of the oral-fecal transmission route.

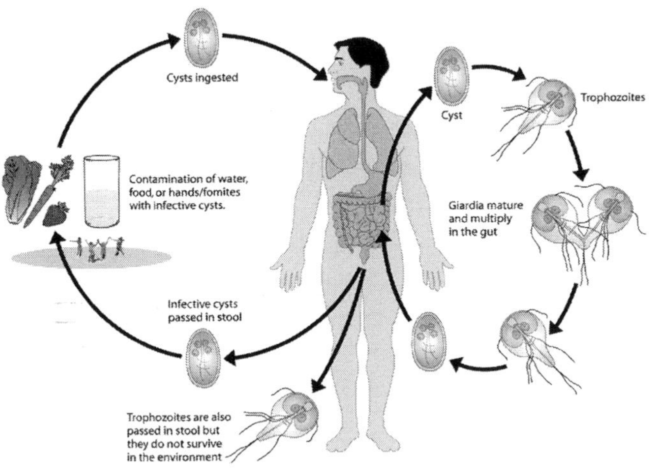

Figure 7.1. Illustration of oral-fecal transmission.

Source: American Society for Microbiology.

The common factors in the fecal-oral route can be summarized as five Fs: fingers, flies, fields, fluids, and food (Rogers, Carolin, Vaught, and Compton, 2011; Ronohardjo and Rastiko, 1982; Sachs, 2001; Sachs and Malaney, 2002). Diseases caused by fecal-oral transmission include diarrhea, typhoid, cholera, polio, and hepatitis (Raut, 2004; Rehm, Mathers, Popova, Thavorncharoensap, Teerawattananon, and Patra, 2009; Rich and Perry, 2011). Although fecal-oral transmission is usually discussed as a route of transmission, it is actually a specification of the entry and exit portals of the pathogen, and can operate across several of the other routes of transmission (Purevdawa, Moon, Baigalmaa, Davaajav, Smith, and Vermund, 1997; Ramesh, Malla, Raju, Sehgal, Ganguly, Mahajan, and Dilawari, 1990). Fecal-oral transmission is primarily considered as an indirect contact route through contaminated food or water (Poundstone, Strathdee, and Celentano, 2004; Pritchett, Thilmany, and Johnson, 2005; Pugliatti, Beghi, Forsgren, Ekman, and Sobocki, 2007). However, it can also operate through direct contact with feces or contaminated body parts, such as through anal sex (Perry and Randolph, 1999; Philipson, 2000; Philipson and Posner, 1996; Pongchaiyakul, Songpattanasilp, and Taechakraichana, 2008). It can also operate through droplet or airborne transmission through the toilet plume from contaminated toilets (Peckham, 2013; Perrings et al., 2002, 2014). The process of transmission may be simple or involve multiple steps. Some examples of routes of fecal-oral transmission include water that has come in contact with feces (for example, due to groundwater pollution from pit latrines) and is then not treated properly before drinking (Pal, Kerorsa, Marami, and Kandi, 2020; Paterson, Otte, Slingenbergh, Wint, and Rogers, 2000; Pearce and Merletti, 2006). It can arise by shaking someone's hand that has been contaminated by stool, changing a child's diapers, working in the garden, or dealing with domestic animals (Ozmen, Kurşun, and Ozcelik, 2005; Paarlberg, Hillberg, Lee, and Mathews, 2008; Paisley, Vraa-Andersen, Dybkjaer, Møller, Christensen, Mousing, and Agger, 1993). There is a risk associated with food that has been prepared in the presence of fecal matter. Additionally, eating soil (geophagia) can accelerate the risks (Oleś, Gudowska-Nowak, and Kleczkowski, 2012; Otte, Nugent, and McLeod, 2004; Ozawa, Portnoy, Getaneh, Clark, Knoll, Bishai, and Patwardhan, 2016). There are certain disease vectors, like houseflies, that help in spreading contamination from inadequate fecal disposal such as open defecation (Narrod, Zinsstag, and Tiongco, 2012; Nascimento and de Oliveira, 2014; O'Brien, Lahue, Caro, and Davidson, 2007). Research has shown that poor or absent hand washing after using the toilet or changing diapers increases risks (Moné, Ibikounlé, Massougbodji, and Mouahid, 2010; Morand, 2004; Moro, Budke, Schantz, Vasquez, Santivanez, and Villavicencio, 2011). Similarly, poor or absent cleaning of anything that has been in contact with feces may lead to this type of transmission (Markos and Abdela, 2016; Martin and Shepherd, 2009; McGuinness, McGlynn, Johnson, MacIntyre, Batty, Burns, and McGinty, 2012). Recently, there has been an acknowledgment of the risk that is associated with sexual practices that may involve oral contact with feces (Krieger, 2001a, b; Lemma, 1969; Liu, Maniadakis, Gray, and Rayner, 2002; López, Torné, Franco, San-Martin, Viayna, Barrull, and Perulero, 2018). Moreover, eating feces, in children, or in a mental disorder called coprophagia will increase the risk of catching diseases in this way (Kim and Goldie, 2008; Klein, Laxminarayan, Smith, and Gilligan, 2007; Klepac, Laxminarayan, and Grenfell, 2011). The next section focuses on propagative transmission.

7.2. PROPAGATIVE TRANSMISSION OF DISEASE EPIDEMICS

Transovarial or transovarian transmission (transmission from parent to offspring via the ovaries) occurs in certain arthropod vectors as they transmit pathogens from parent arthropod to offspring arthropod (Jenkins, Baingana,

Ahmad, McDaid, and Atun, 2011; Johnson, Alvarez-Pasquin, Bijl, Franco, Gaillat, Clara, and Weinke, 2015). For instance, *Rickettsia rickettsii*, carried within ticks, is passed on from parent to offspring tick by transovarial transmission (Howe, Häsler, and Stärk, 2013; Howe et al., 2012). In contrast, Rickettsia prowazekii is not passed on by transovarian transmission because it kills the vector that carries it which is the human louse (Hart and Halden, 2020; Häsler, Howe, and Stärk, 2011; Henschke, Kamper, and Maher, 2015; Hochberg, 1992). This is the mechanism by which many Rickettsiae are maintained in their arthropod hosts through generations, which occurs also in Aedes mosquito vector of the yellow fever virus and in phlebotomine sandflies that transmit pappataci fever (Foxman, 2002; Garner, Whan, Gard, and Phillips, 2001; Gayle and Hill, 2001; Gottstein, Pozio, and Nöckler, 2009). The mechanism of propagative transmission is summarized in Figure 7.2.

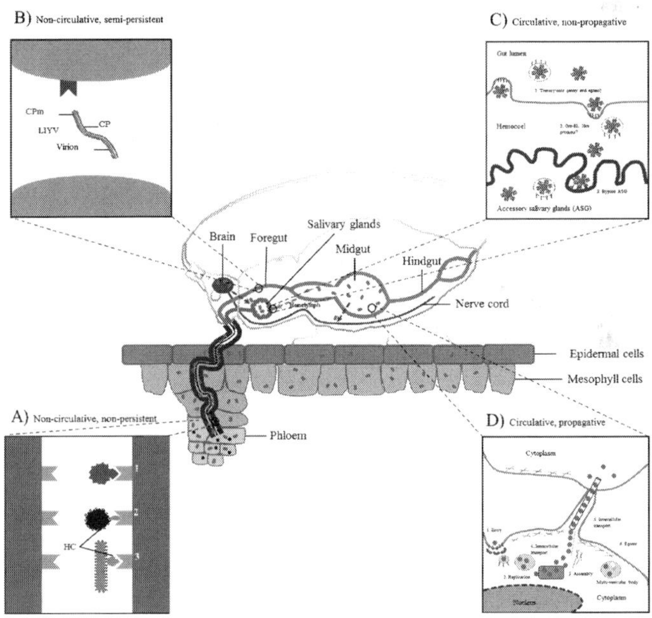

Figure 7.2. Propagative transmission of disease.

Source: MDPI.

Richard Dawkins (1999, p.222) in "*The Extended Phenotype*" suggests that bacterial endosymbionts of insects which are transmitted transovarially share an interest in the success of their host's gametes as well as the survival of their host's body (Fenichel, 2013; Fenichel et al., 2011; Fogel, 1994).

Hence, the interest of the host genes and parasite genes might not be quite identical (Espinoza, Terashima, Herrera-Velit, and Marcos, 2010; Ezzati, Vander Hoorn, Lawes, Leach, James, Lopez, and Murray, 2005). However, they would be very much closer than the case of fluke and snail where host and parasite have different means of propagation into the next generation, and therefore more divergent interests (Eaton and Groopman, 2013; Eckelman, Sherman, and MacNeill, 2018; Egger, 2011; Elbe, 2007; Ernst and Hay, 1994).

Transstadial transmission occurs when a pathogen remains with the vector from one life stage ("stadium") to the next (Daily and Ehrlich, 1996; Deogaonkar, Hutubessy, Van Der Putten, Evers, and Jit, 2012; Dorn, 1992; Ducrotoy, Bertu, Ocholi, Gusi, Bryssinckx, Welburn, and Moriyon, 2014). For example, the bacteria Borrelia burgdorferi, the causative agent for Lyme disease, infects the tick vector as a larva, and the infection is maintained when it molts to a nymph and later develops as an adult (Chen, Li, Hsieh, Chang, Lee, Lee, and Ko, 2012; Conover, Pitt, Kessler, DuBow, and Sanborn, 1995; Crump, Murdoch, and Baker, 2001). This type of transmission is seen in other parasites like viruses or Rickettsia. In addition to ticks, mites are another common vector (Casamassimo, Thikkurissy, Edelstein, and Maiorini, 2009; Castro, Wilson, and Bloom, 2017). Some sources consider transstadial transmission a type of horizontal transmission (Bwire, Munier, Ouedraogo, Heyerdahl, Komakech, Kagirita, and Makumbi, 2017; Canali, Aragrande, Angheben, Capelli, Drigo, Gobbi, and Cassini, 2020). Yet, other sources consider it vertical or partial vertical transmission (Buckley, 1984; Budke, Jiamin, Qian, and Torgerson, 2005; Bundy, Arámbulo III, and Grey, 1983; Buzby and Roberts, 2009). Transstadial blockage could be considered the opposite of transstadial transmission, where the parasite cannot be carried over from one life stage to the next (Borghol, Suderman, McArdle, Racine, Hallett, Pembrey, and Szyf, 2012; Brandes, 2008; Brown, Lipscomb, and Snyder, 2001). For example, viruses that undergo transstadial blockage will have decreased infectivity in molting insects (Bonds, Keenan, Rohani, and Sachs, 2010; Boni, Galvani, Wickelgren, and Malani, 2013; Bonovas and Nikolopoulos, 2012).

Viruses are known to infect both plant cells and animal cells (Bergevoet, Van Schaik, Veling, Backus, and Franken, 2009; Binder, 1988; Bolos, Bacarea, and Marusteri, 2011). Since viruses are obligate intracellular parasites, they must develop direct methods of transmission, between hosts, in order to survive (Bausch and Schwarz, 2014; Bausch et al., 2001; Benner, Carabin, Sánchez-Serrano, Budke, and Carmena, 2010). The mobility of animals increases the mechanisms of viral transmission that have evolved, whereas plants remain immobile and thus plant viruses must rely on environmental factors to be transmitted between hosts (Arredondo and Zúñiga, 2006; Backer, van Roermund, Fischer, van Asseldonk, and Bergevoet, 2015; Bartsch, Hotez, Hertenstein, Diemert, Zapf, Bottazzi, and Lee, 2016). The structural differences between plant and animal cells have resulted in a variety of transmission routes being exploited, enabling the virus to be passed between different host plants (Armelagos, Brown, and Turner, 2005; Arokiasamy and Krishnan, 1994; Arora, 2001, 2005; Arredondo and Zúñiga, 2004). The main difference, from the point of view of a virus, is the cell wall (Amuna and Zotor, 2008; Aral, Holmes, Padian, and Cates, 1996; Arbabi, Nezami, Hooshyar, and Delavari, 2018). This forms a tough barrier between the intracellular components and the extracellular environment, which has to be penetrated (Acemoglu and Johnson, 2007; Adda, 2016; Alloul, Sauriol, Kennedy, Laurier, Tessier, Novosel, and Contandriopoulos, 1998).

These differences, combined with the fact that plants are immobile, have resulted in plant viruses relying on the wind and soil to transmit seeds as well as vectors (Abegunde and Stanciole, 2008; Abramowitz, Lacau Saint Guily, Moyal-Barracco, Bergeron, Borne, Dahlab, and Bénard, 2018). Vectors either transmit the virus propagative transmission, which results in an amplification of the virus by replication within the cells of the vector, or non-propagative transmission which simply carries the virus between the plants without viral replication. Common vectors include Bacteria, Fungi, Nematodes, arthropods, and arachnids (Ozmen, Kurşun, and Ozcelik, 2005; Paarlberg, Hillberg, Lee, and Mathews, 2008; Paisley, Vraa-Andersen, Dybkjaer, Møller, Christensen, Mousing, and Agger, 1993). Furthermore, human intervention, including grafting and experimental mechanical damage, physically damages the cell wall, contributes to the array of transmission routes (Bonds, Keenan, Rohani, and Sachs, 2010; Boni, Galvani, Wickelgren, and Malani, 2013; Bonovas and Nikolopoulos, 2012). The virus commonly uses these methods to be passed from one host to another (Espinoza, Terashima, Herrera-Velit, and Marcos, 2010; Ezzati, Vander Hoorn, Lawes, Leach, James, Lopez, and Murray, 2005). However, the virus is dependent upon physical damage, generated naturally by the wind and feeding of vectors or by human intervention (Buckley, 1984; Budke, Jiamin, Qian, and Torgerson, 2005; Bundy, Arámbulo III, and Grey, 1983; Buzby and Roberts, 2009). Viral infections often develop into systemic infections as a means of transmission (Bwire, Munier, Ouedraogo,

Heyerdahl, Komakech, Kagirita, and Makumbi, 2017; Canali, Aragrande, Angheben, Capelli, Drigo, Gobbi, and Cassini, 2020). The virus often infects many tissues, if not the whole plant, where it can continue to replicate (Pal, Kerorsa, Marami, and Kandi, 2020; Paterson, Otte, Slingenbergh, Wint, and Rogers, 2000; Pearce and Merletti, 2006). There are a variety of methods the virus can use to spread throughout the organism, but the most common route uses the vascular system, otherwise known as the xylem and phloem, and the plasmodesmata, which interconnect adjacent cells (Yi-Xin and Manderson, 2005; Zadoks, 2008; Zhan, Li, Wang, Sun, Geng, Xiong, and de Hoog, 2015; Zhang, Song, Cai, and Zhou, 2008). Nevertheless, the rigidity of the cell wall of plant cells, not only poses a problem for transmission of the viruses between different plant hosts, but also acts to prevent viral transmission between cells (Jenkins, Baingana, Ahmad, McDaid, and Atun, 2011; Johnson, Alvarez-Pasquin, Bijl, Franco, Gaillat, Clara, and Weinke, 2015). Consequently, the virus must modify the plasmodesmata as they, themselves, are too large to fit through the small and tightly regulated plant structure (Abegunde and Stanciole, 2008; Abramowitz, Lacau Saint Guily, Moyal-Barracco, Bergeron, Borne, Dahlab, and Bénard, 2018). There are again a variety of mechanisms used for this, which have evolved for different viruses (Kim and Goldie, 2008; Klein, Laxminarayan, Smith, and Gilligan, 2007; Klepac, Laxminarayan, and Grenfell, 2011). The main mechanisms involve expressing proteins which coat the virus and interact with the structure of the plasmodesmata (Chen, Li, Hsieh, Chang, Lee, Lee, and Ko, 2012; Conover, Pitt, Kessler, DuBow, and Sanborn, 1995; Crump, Murdoch, and Baker, 2001). The array of proteins expressed by the different viruses may act differently, but all achieve a similar goal, passage between adjacent cells (Weycker, Edelsberg, Oster, and Tino, 2005; Wu, Perrings, Kinzig, Collins, Minteer, and Daszak, 2017; Yach, Stuckler, and Brownell, 2006). This chapter will close with a review of vertical transmission of diseases.

7.3. VERTICAL TRANSMISSION OF DISEASE EPIDEMICS

A vertically transmitted infection is an infection caused by pathogens (such as bacteria and viruses) that use mother-to-child transmission, that is, transmission directly from the mother to an embryo, fetus, or baby during pregnancy or childbirth (Perry and Randolph, 1999; Philipson, 2000; Philipson and Posner, 1996; Pongchaiyakul, Songpattanasilp, and Taechakraichana, 2008). It can occur when the mother has a pre-existing disease or becomes infected during pregnancy. Nutritional deficiencies may exacerbate the risks of perinatal infections (Uusküla, Müürsepp, Kawai, Raag, Jürisson, and Pillsbury, 2013; Vanni, Karnon, Madan, White, Edmunds, Foss, and Legood, 2011). Bacteria, viruses, and other organisms are able to be passed from mother to child (St George, 1986; Steben and Duarte-Franco, 2007; Stehr-Green and Schantz, 1987; Stuckler, 2008; Stuckler and Siegel, 2011). Figure 7.3 represents an illustration of the vertical transmission of HTLV-1.

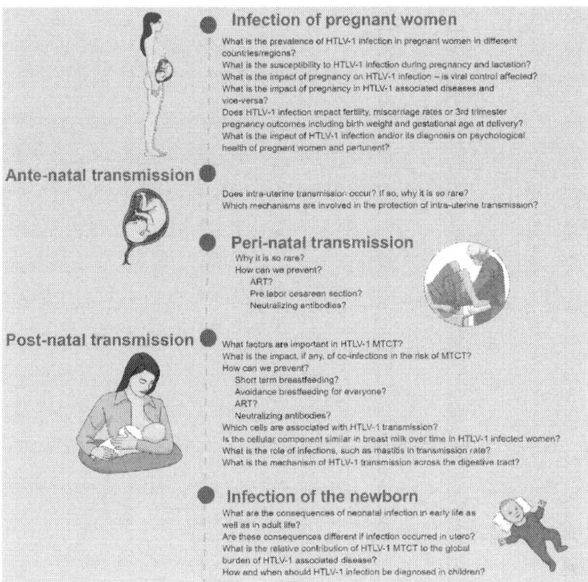

Figure 7.3. Example of vertical transmission of HTLV-1.

Source: Frontiers.

Several vertically transmitted infections are included in the TORCH complex in which encompasses:

- T-toxoplasmosis from Toxoplasma gondii;
- O-other infections including Parvovirus B19, Coxsackievirus, Chickenpox (caused by varicella-zoster virus), Chlamydia, and HIV;
- R-rubella;
- C-cytomegalovirus;
- H-herpes simplex virus-2 or neonatal herpes simplex.

Hepatitis B may also be classified as a vertically transmitted infection (Acemoglu and Johnson, 2007; Adda, 2016; Alloul, Sauriol, Kennedy, Laurier, Tessier, Novosel, and Contandriopoulos, 1998). The hepatitis B virus is large and does not cross the placenta (Amuna and Zotor, 2008; Aral, Holmes, Padian, and Cates, 1996; Arbabi, Nezami, Hooshyar, and Delavari, 2018). Hence, it cannot infect the fetus unless breaks in the maternal-fetal barrier have occurred, but such breaks can occur in bleeding during childbirth or amniocentesis (Krieger, 2001a, b; Lemma, 1969; Liu, Maniadakis, Gray, and Rayner, 2002; López, Torné, Franco, San-Martin, Viayna, Barrull, and Perulero, 2018). The TORCH complex was originally considered to consist of the four conditions mentioned above, with the "TO" referring to Toxoplasma (Armelagos, Brown, and Turner, 2005; Arokiasamy and Krishnan, 1994; Arora, 2001, 2005; Arredondo and Zúñiga, 2004). The four-term form is still used in many modern references and the capitalization "ToRCH" is sometimes used in these contexts (Poundstone, Strathdee, and Celentano, 2004; Pritchett, Thilmany, and Johnson, 2005; Pugliatti, Beghi, Forsgren, Ekman, and Sobocki, 2007). The acronym has also been listed as TORCHES, for TOxoplasmosis, Rubella, Cytomegalovirus, HErpes simplex, and Syphilis (Suhrcke, Stuckler, Suk, Desai, Senek, McKee, and Rechel, 2011; Šumilo, Bormane, Asokliene, Vasilenko, Golovljova, Avsic-Zupanc, and Randolph, 2008).

A further expansion of this acronym, CHEAPTORCHES, was proposed by Ford-Jones and Kellner in 1995 including:

- C-chickenpox and shingles;
- H-hepatitis, C, (D), E;
- E-enteroviruses;
- A-AIDS (HIV infection);
- P-parvovirus B19 (produces hydrops fetalis secondary to aplastic anemia);
- T-toxoplasmosis;
- Other (group B streptococci, Listeria, Candida, and Lyme disease);
- R-rubella;
- C-cytomegalovirus;
- H-herpes simplex;

- E-everything else sexually transmitted (gonorrhea, Chlamydia infection, *Ureaplasma urealyticum*, and human papillomavirus);
- S-Syphilis.

The signs and symptoms of a vertically transmitted infection depend on the individual pathogen (Bergevoet, Van Schaik, Veling, Backus, and Franken, 2009; Binder, 1988; Bolos, Bacarea, and Marusteri, 2011). In the mother, it may cause subtle signs such as an influenza-like illness, or possibly no symptoms at all. In such cases, the effects may be seen first at birth (Arredondo and Zúñiga, 2006; Backer, van Roermund, Fischer, van Asseldonk, and Bergevoet, 2015; Bartsch, Hotez, Hertenstein, Diemert, Zapf, Bottazzi, and Lee, 2016). Symptoms of a vertically transmitted infection may include fever and flu-like symptoms (Howe, Häsler, and Stärk, 2013; Howe et al., 2012). The newborn is often small for gestational age (Raut, 2004; Rehm, Mathers, Popova, Thavorncharoensap, Teerawattananon, and Patra, 2009; Rich and Perry, 2011). A petechial rash on the skin may be present, with small reddish or purplish spots due to bleeding from capillaries under the skin (Hart and Halden, 2020; Häsler, Howe, and Stärk, 2011; Henschke, Kamper, and Maher, 2015; Hochberg, 1992. An enlarged liver and spleen (hepatosplenomegaly) is common, as is jaundice (Markos and Abdela, 2016; Martin and Shepherd, 2009; McGuinness, McGlynn, Johnson, MacIntyre, Batty, Burns, and McGinty, 2012). However, jaundice is less common in hepatitis B because a newborn's immune system is not developed well enough to mount a response against liver cells, as would normally be the cause of jaundice in an older child or adult (Foxman, 2002; Garner, Whan, Gard, and Phillips, 2001; Gayle and Hill, 2001; Gottstein, Pozio, and Nöckler, 2009). Hearing impairment, eye problems, mental retardation, autism, and death can be caused by vertically transmitted infections (Moné, Ibikounlé, Massougbodji, and Mouahid, 2010; Morand, 2004; Moro, Budke, Schantz, Vasquez, Santivanez, and Villavicencio, 2011). The genetic conditions of Aicardi-Goutieres syndrome are possibly present in a similar manner (Eaton and Groopman, 2013; Eckelman, Sherman, and MacNeill, 2018; Egger, 2011; Elbe, 2007; Ernst and Hay, 1994).

The main routes of transmission of vertically transmitted infections are across the placenta (transplacental) and across the female reproductive tract during childbirth (Oleś, Gudowska-Nowak, and Kleczkowski, 2012; Otte, Nugent, and McLeod, 2004; Ozawa, Portnoy, Getaneh, Clark, Knoll, Bishai, and Patwardhan, 2016). Transmission is also possible by breaks in the maternal-fetal barrier such by amniocentesis or major trauma (Rogers, Carolin, Vaught, and Compton, 2011; Ronohardjo and Rastiko, 1982; Sachs,

2001; Sachs and Malaney, 2002). The embryo and fetus have little or no immune function (Bausch and Schwarz, 2014; Bausch et al., 2001; Benner, Carabin, Sánchez-Serrano, Budke, and Carmena, 2010). They depend on the immune function of their mother (Purevdawa, Moon, Baigalmaa, Davaajav, Smith, and Vermund, 1997; Ramesh, Malla, Raju, Sehgal, Ganguly, Mahajan, and Dilawari, 1990). Several pathogens can cross the placenta and cause perinatal infection (Borghol, Suderman, McArdle, Racine, Hallett, Pembrey, and Szyf, 2012; Brandes, 2008; Brown, Lipscomb, and Snyder, 2001). Often, microorganisms that produce minor illness in the mother are very dangerous for the developing embryo or fetus (Tapia, 2003; Torgerson and Dowling, 2001; Torgerson, Carmona, and Bonifacino, 2000; Uddin Khan, Atanasova, Krueger, Ramirez, and Gray, 2013). This can result in spontaneous abortion or major developmental disorders (Saleha, 1991; Sibert, Rigaud, Delavierre, and Labat, 2010; Skrepnek and Skrepnek, 2004; Sloane, 2009; Sockett, 1993). For many infections, the baby is more at risk at particular stages of pregnancy (Peckham, 2013; Perrings et al., 2002, 2014). Problems related to perinatal infection are not always directly noticeable (Daily and Ehrlich, 1996; Deogaonkar, Hutubessy, Van Der Putten, Evers, and Jit, 2012; Dorn, 1992; Ducrotoy, Bertu, Ocholi, Gusi, Bryssinckx, Welburn, and Moriyon, 2014).

Babies can also become infected by their mothers during birth (Fenichel, 2013; Fenichel et al., 2011; Fogel, 1994). Some infectious agents may be transmitted to the embryo or fetus in the uterus, while passing through the birth canal, or even shortly after birth (Narrod, Zinsstag, and Tiongco, 2012; Nascimento and de Oliveira, 2014; O'Brien, Lahue, Caro, and Davidson, 2007). The distinction is important because when transmission is primarily during or after birth, medical intervention can help prevent infections in the infant (Casamassimo, Thikkurissy, Edelstein, and Maiorini, 2009; Castro, Wilson, and Bloom, 2017). During birth, babies are exposed to maternal blood, body fluids, and to the maternal genital tract without the placental barrier intervening (Abegunde and Stanciole, 2008; Abramowitz, Lacau Saint Guily, Moyal-Barracco, Bergeron, Borne, Dahlab, and Bénard, 2018). Because of this, blood-borne microorganisms (hepatitis B, HIV), organisms associated with sexually transmitted diseases (e.g., Neisseria gonorrhea and Chlamydia trachomatis), and normal fauna of the genitourinary tract (e.g., Candida albicans) are among those commonly seen in infection of newborns (Acemoglu and Johnson, 2007; Adda, 2016; Alloul, Sauriol, Kennedy, Laurier, Tessier, Novosel, and Contandriopoulos, 1998).

In the spectrum of optimal virulence, vertical transmission tends to evolve benign symbiosis, so is a critical concept for evolutionary medicine (Amuna and Zotor, 2008; Aral, Holmes, Padian, and Cates, 1996; Arbabi, Nezami, Hooshyar, and Delavari, 2018). Because a pathogen's ability to pass from mother to child depends significantly on the hosts' ability to reproduce, pathogens' transmissibility tends to be inversely related to their virulence (Armelagos, Brown, and Turner, 2005; Arokiasamy and Krishnan, 1994; Arora, 2001, 2005; Arredondo and Zúñiga, 2004). In other words, as pathogens become more harmful to, and thus decrease the reproduction rate of, their host organism, they are less likely to be passed on to the hosts' offspring, since they will have fewer offspring (Arredondo and Zúñiga, 2006; Backer, van Roermund, Fischer, van Asseldonk, and Bergevoet, 2015; Bartsch, Hotez, Hertenstein, Diemert, Zapf, Bottazzi, and Lee, 2016). Although HIV is sometimes transmitted through perinatal transmission, its virulence can be accounted for because its primary mode of transmission is not vertical (Bausch and Schwarz, 2014; Bausch et al., 2001; Benner, Carabin, Sánchez-Serrano, Budke, and Carmena, 2010). Moreover, medicine has further decreased the frequency of vertical transmission of HIV (Bergevoet, Van Schaik, Veling, Backus, and Franken, 2009; Binder, 1988; Bolos, Bacarea, and Marusteri, 2011). The incidence of perinatal HIV cases in the United States has declined as a result of the implementation of recommendations on HIV counseling and voluntary testing practices and the use of zidovudine therapy by providers to reduce perinatal HIV transmission (Bonds, Keenan, Rohani, and Sachs, 2010; Boni, Galvani, Wickelgren, and Malani, 2013; Bonovas and Nikolopoulos, 2012).

The price paid in the evolution of symbiosis is significant (Borghol, Suderman, McArdle, Racine, Hallett, Pembrey, and Szyf, 2012; Brandes, 2008; Brown, Lipscomb, and Snyder, 2001). For many generations, almost all cases of vertical transmission continue to be pathological. This is particularly true if any other routes of transmission exist (Buckley, 1984; Budke, Jiamin, Qian, and Torgerson, 2005; Bundy, Arámbulo III, and Grey, 1983; Buzby and Roberts, 2009). Many generations of random mutation and selection are needed to evolve symbiosis (Bwire, Munier, Ouedraogo, Heyerdahl, Komakech, Kagirita, and Makumbi, 2017; Canali, Aragrande, Angheben, Capelli, Drigo, Gobbi, and Cassini, 2020). During this time, the vast majority of vertical transmission cases exhibit the initial virulence. In dual inheritance theory, vertical transmission refers to the passing of cultural traits from parents to children (Casamassimo, Thikkurissy, Edelstein, and Maiorini, 2009; Castro, Wilson, and Bloom, 2017). When physical examination of the newborn shows signs of a vertically transmitted infection, the examiner may test blood, urine, and spinal fluid for evidence of the infections listed above (Chen, Li, Hsieh, Chang, Lee, Lee, and Ko, 2012; Conover, Pitt, Kessler, DuBow, and Sanborn, 1995; Crump, Murdoch, and Baker, 2001). Diagnosis can be confirmed by culture of one of the specific pathogens or by increased levels of IgM against the pathogen (Daily, and Ehrlich, 1996; Deogaonkar, Hutubessy, Van Der Putten, Evers, and Jit, 2012; Dorn, 1992; Ducrotoy, Bertu, Ocholi, Gusi, Bryssinckx, Welburn, and Moriyon, 2014).

A vertically transmitted infection can be called a perinatal infection if it is transmitted in the perinatal period (Eaton and Groopman, 2013; Eckelman, Sherman, and MacNeill, 2018; Egger, 2011; Elbe, 2007; Ernst and Hay, 1994). This starts at gestational ages between 22 and 28 weeks (with regional variations in the definition) and ending seven completed days after birth (Espinoza, Terashima, Herrera-Velit, and Marcos, 2010; Ezzati, Vander Hoorn, Lawes, Leach, James, Lopez, and Murray, 2005). The term congenital infection can be used if the vertically transmitted infection persists after childbirth (Fenichel, 2013; Fenichel et al., 2011; Fogel, 1994). Some vertically transmitted infections, such as toxoplasmosis and syphilis, can be effectively treated with antibiotics if the mother is diagnosed early in her pregnancy (Foxman, 2002; Garner, Whan, Gard, and Phillips, 2001; Gayle and Hill, 2001; Gottstein, Pozio, and Nöckler, 2009).

Many viral vertically transmitted infections have no effective treatment. However, some (notably rubella and varicella-zoster) can be prevented by vaccinating the mother prior to pregnancy (Hart and Halden, 2020; Häsler, Howe, and Stärk, 2011; Henschke, Kamper, and Maher, 2015; Hochberg, 1992). Pregnant women living in malaria-endemic areas are candidates for malaria prophylaxis (Howe, Häsler, and Stärk, 2013; Howe et al., 2012). It clinically improves the anemia and parasitemia of the pregnant women, and birthweight in their infants (Jenkins, Baingana, Ahmad, McDaid, and Atun, 2011; Johnson, Alvarez-Pasquin, Bijl, Franco, Gaillat, Clara, and Weinke, 2015). If the mother has active herpes simplex (as may be suggested by a pap test), delivery by Caesarean section can prevent the newborn from contact, and consequent infection, with this virus (Kim and Goldie, 2008; Klein, Laxminarayan, Smith, and Gilligan, 2007; Klepac, Laxminarayan, and Grenfell, 2011). IgG2 antibody may play a crucial role in the prevention of intrauterine infections and extensive research is going on for developing IgG2-based therapies for treatment and vaccination (Krieger, 2001a, b; Lemma, 1969; Liu, Maniadakis, Gray, and Rayner, 2002; López, Torné,

Franco, San-Martin, Viayna, Barrull, and Perulero, 2018). Each type of vertically transmitted infection has a different prognosis (Markos and Abdela, 2016; Martin and Shepherd, 2009; McGuinness, McGlynn, Johnson, Macintyre, Batty, Burns, and McGinty, 2012). The stage of the pregnancy at the time of infection also can change the effect on the newborn (Moné, Ibikounlé, Massougbodji, and Mouahid, 2010; Morand, 2004; Moro, Budke, Schantz, Vasquez, Santivanez, and Villavicencio, 2011).

CHAPTER 7 SUMMARY

Chapter 6 and 7 of this book have explored a range of transmission modalities for disease epidemicsDisease epidemics including fecal-oral, horizontal, vertical, and propagative. It is important to understand these modalities because they inform all the decisions that are taken to prevent, stall, or even eradicate certain disease epidemicsDisease epidemics. The last chapter in this book will focus on the overall impact of disease epidemicsDisease epidemics on a community.

Chapter

8

Impact of Disease Epidemics

CONTENTS

Disease epidemics impact on communities in different and multi-faceted ways. Although this book has primarily highlighted the economic impact, the nature of the overall impact can be social, economic, political, environmental, and even legal. These dynamics are explored in the final chapter of the book in order to emphasize the fact that behind all the clinical diagnoses and treatments; epidemics or even pandemics have real consequences for humanity. Indeed, this final chapter may be seen as a call for action, both preventative and responsive, in order to mitigate against some of these impacts. We will begin the chapter by exploring the politics of Disease epidemics.

8.1. POLITICS OF DISEASE EPIDEMICS

Over the past few decades, disease outbreaks have become increasingly frequent and widespread (Narrod, Zinsstag, and Tiongco, 2012; Nascimento and de Oliveira, 2014; O'Brien, Lahue, Caro, and Davidson, 2007). The epicenters of these outbreaks have differed, and could be linked to different economic contexts (Oleś, Gudowska-Nowak, and Kleczkowski, 2012; Otte, Nugent, and McLeod, 2004; Ozawa, Portnoy, Getaneh, Clark, Knoll, Bishai, and Patwardhan, 2016). Arguably, the responses to these outbreaks have been "political" and inherently burdensome to marginalized populations (Ozmen, Kurşun, and Ozcelik, 2005; Paarlberg, Hillberg, Lee, and Mathews, 2008; Paisley, Vraa-Andersen, Dybkjaer, Møller, Christensen, Mousing, and Agger, 1993). Key lessons can be learned from exploring the narratives about the different epidemics in varying income settings (Pal, Kerorsa, Marami, and Kandi, 2020; Paterson, Otte, Slingenbergh, Wint, and Rogers, 2000; Pearce and Merletti, 2006). Various themes of the politics of epidemics are prominent in existing literature (Peckham, 2013; Perrings et al., 2002, 2014). The narratives demonstrated the influence of power in whose narratives and what narratives are presented in the literature (Perry and Randolph, 1999; Philipson, 2000; Philipson and Posner, 1996; Pongchaiyakul, Songpattanasilp, and Taechakraichana, 2008). As the leading global hegemony, the USA tends to provide funding for global health security, which is linked to the outbreaks of pandemics (see Figure 8.1).

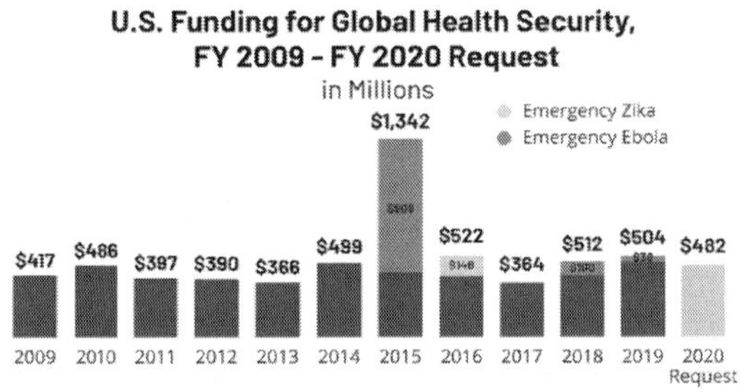

Figure 8.1. Health security expenditures and epidemics.

Source: Kaiser Family Foundation.

While marginalized populations were reported to have borne the brunt of all disease outbreaks in the different contexts, the prevalence of their narratives within existing literature is limited (Poundstone, Strathdee, and Celentano, 2004; Pritchett, Thilmany, and Johnson, 2005; Pugliatti, Beghi, Forsgren, Ekman, and Sobocki, 2007). Regardless of income setting, there is a need to give voice to the most marginalized communities during an epidemic (Purevdawa, Moon, Baigalmaa, Davaajav, Smith, and Vermund, 1997; Ramesh, Malla, Raju, Sehgal, Ganguly, Mahajan, and Dilawari, 1990). The experiences and narratives of those most vulnerable to an epidemic to be represented in the literature (Raut, 2004; Rehm, Mathers, Popova, Thavorncharoensap, Teerawattananon, and Patra, 2009; Rich and Perry, 2011). This could contribute to the mitigation of some of the negative impact of politics in epidemics (Rogers, Carolin, Vaught, and Compton, 2011; Ronohardjo and Rastiko, 1982; Sachs, 2001; Sachs and Malaney, 2002). Several key themes emerge when examining scholarly narratives about the politics of epidemics (Saleha, 1991; Sibert, Rigaud, Delavierre, and Labat, 2010; Skrepnek and Skrepnek, 2004; Sloane, 2009; Sockett, 1993). These themes include the socioeconomic distribution of disease, decision-making in research and development, the credibility of evidence that informs response pathways, and attribution of responsibility for causing the outbreak and determining who is responsible for responding (St George, 1986; Steben and Duarte-Franco, 2007; Stehr-Green and Schantz, 1987; Stuckler, 2008; Stuckler and Siegel, 2011).

While the literature presents obviously competing narratives that explain disease outbreaks, a close examination of these reveals a high prevalence of certain narratives, which reflect the influence of power and privilege (Suhrcke, Stuckler, Suk, Desai, Senek, McKee, and Rechel, 2011; Šumilo, Bormane, Asokliene, Vasilenko, Golovljova, Avsic-Zupanc, and Randolph, 2008). Hence, some of the literature has called for increased representation of the narratives from the most marginalized populations who bear the brunt of epidemics, in the scholarly literature (Tapia, 2003; Torgerson and Dowling, 2001; Torgerson, Carmona, and Bonifacino, 2000; Uddin Khan, Atanasova, Krueger, Ramirez, and Gray, 2013). Many of the research exercises focusing on epidemics end up re-marginalizing the poorest and most vulnerable, ironically the most affected by these epidemics (Uusküla, Müürsepp, Kawai, Raag, Jürisson, and Pillsbury, 2013; Vanni, Karnon, Madan, White, Edmunds, Foss, and Legood, 2011). For example, the study population and the research beneficiaries often lack transparency, are also dominated by the most powerful (Weycker, Edelsberg, Oster, and Tino, 2005; Wu, Perrings, Kinzig, Collins, Minteer, and Daszak, 2017; Yach, Stuckler, and Brownell, 2006). The case of swine flu, dubbed the "pandemic that never really was" demonstrates the potential consequences of private and uncommunicated decision-making processes in research and development (Yi-Xin and Manderson, 2005; Zadoks, 2008; Zhan, Li, Wang, Sun, Geng, Xiong, and de Hoog, 2015; Zhang, Song, Cai, and Zhou, 2008).

In the case of the swine flu misrepresentation, allegedly scientists conducting research and advising the World Health Organization (WHO) on the virus were compensated by drug companies (Casamassimo, Thikkurissy, Edelstein, and Maiorini, 2009; Castro, Wilson, and Bloom, 2017). This may have introduced a bias and is indicative of the general failure to account for the narratives and experiences of those that are most affected by disease epidemicsDisease epidemics (Narrod, Zinsstag, and Tiongco, 2012; Nascimento and de Oliveira, 2014; O'Brien, Lahue, Caro, and Davidson, 2007). By increasing fear of a global pandemic, scientific research funded by pharmaceutical companies justified the stockpiling of anti-viral supplies, thus increasing their vaccine sales; a case in point demonstrating how the research process can be corrupted (Fenichel, 2013; Fenichel et al., 2011; Fogel, 1994).

Fear mongering has been criticized in the literature, since it has the potential to distort the evidence, which should guide credible decision-making (Daily, and Ehrlich, 1996; Deogaonkar, Hutubessy, Van Der Putten, Evers, and Jit, 2012; Dorn, 1992; Ducrotoy, Bertu, Ocholi, Gusi, Bryssinckx, Welburn, and Moriyon, 2014). In recent times, there have been deniers for virtually all epidemics meaning that initial responses have been hampered due to resistance (Peckham, 2013; Perrings et al., 2002, 2014). The scientific conspiracy theory is very much a growing niche on the internet where irresponsible and unsubstantiated accusations can be made against anyone (Saleha, 1991; Sibert, Rigaud, Delavierre, and Labat, 2010; Skrepnek and Skrepnek, 2004; Sloane, 2009; Sockett, 1993). It is therefore critical to assess the credibility and quality of the evidence that is being used to inform the response to epidemics around the world, particularly in light of the complicated and often problematic relationship between the academic and industry (Tapia, 2003; Torgerson and Dowling, 2001; Torgerson, Carmona, and Bonifacino, 2000; Uddin Khan, Atanasova, Krueger, Ramirez, and Gray, 2013). In determining the credibility of evidence, consideration should be given to the legitimacy and authority of its producers (Borghol, Suderman, McArdle, Racine, Hallett, Pembrey, and Szyf, 2012; Brandes, 2008; Brown, Lipscomb, and Snyder, 2001).

Existing literature identifies discourse about the attribution of responsibility. Many wonder who is to blame for the outbreak and who should respond (Purevdawa, Moon, Baigalmaa, Davaajav, Smith, and Vermund, 1997; Ramesh, Malla, Raju, Sehgal, Ganguly, Mahajan, and Dilawari, 1990). In the case of the Corona Virus, some prominent US politicians have attempted to shift the blame to China (Bausch and Schwarz, 2014; Bausch et al., 2001; Benner, Carabin, Sánchez-Serrano, Budke, and Carmena, 2010). As a consequence, some countries have withdrawn or have threatened to withdraw from the WHO, a decision that has been greeted with displeasure and horror by public health experts (Rogers, Carolin, Vaught, and Compton, 2011; Ronohardjo and Rastiko, 1982; Sachs, 2001; Sachs and Malaney, 2002). There is literature that has assigned the blame and responsibility for disease epidemicsDisease epidemics to people's cultures (Oleś, Gudowska-Nowak, and Kleczkowski, 2012; Otte, Nugent, and McLeod, 2004; Ozawa, Portnoy, Getaneh, Clark, Knoll, Bishai, and Patwardhan, 2016). This in effect oversimplifies complex issues that result from complex processes, such as globalization, climate change, and global economics (Eaton and Groopman, 2013; Eckelman, Sherman, and MacNeill, 2018; Egger, 2011; Elbe, 2007; Ernst and Hay, 1994). This kind of narrative reflects the politics of blame, which typically attributes responsibility for the sources of the outbreak to a cultural minority group (Moné, Ibikounlé, Massougbodji, and Mouahid, 2010; Morand, 2004; Moro, Budke, Schantz, Vasquez, Santivanez, and Villavicencio, 2011). Such attitudes simultaneously neglect the influence of colonialism and the social determinants of health, including overcrowding, poor sanitation, and poverty that increase these people's vulnerability (Foxman, 2002; Garner, Whan, Gard, and Phillips, 2001; Gayle and Hill,

2001; Gottstein, Pozio, and Nöckler, 2009). For example, the systematic colonization and recolonization of African governments has a role to play in making African people more susceptible to disease epidemicsDisease epidemics (Markos and Abdela, 2016; Martin and Shepherd, 2009; McGuinness, McGlynn, Johnson, MacIntyre, Batty, Burns, and McGinty, 2012). That is not to diminish the responsibility of local communities and their accountability for the decisions they do or do not take (Hart and Halden, 2020; Häsler, Howe, and Stärk, 2011; Henschke, Kamper, and Maher, 2015; Hochberg, 1992).

Given these sociopolitical issues that characterize epidemics, a comparative analysis of the narratives on the politics of epidemics is relevant (Raut, 2004; Rehm, Mathers, Popova, Thavorncharoensap, Teerawattananon, and Patra, 2009; Rich and Perry, 2011). To date, most of the narratives in the scholarly literature on the politics of epidemics have considered one epidemic in one context (Howe, Häsler, and Stärk, 2013; Howe et al., 2012). However, the narratives of disease epidemics may vary depending on the kind and context of the epidemic (Arredondo and Zúñiga, 2006; Backer, van Roermund, Fischer, van Asseldonk, and Bergevoet, 2015; Bartsch, Hotez, Hertenstein, Diemert, Zapf, Bottazzi, and Lee, 2016). Politics is very much part of the context and could impact on virtually all the processes that take place during the epidemics (Bergevoet, Van Schaik, Veling, Backus, and Franken, 2009; Binder, 1988; Bolos, Bacarea, and Marusteri, 2011). With fears of global health epidemics (of reemerging infectious diseases) having escalated over the past few decades, we must ask how we understand the diverse responses to such outbreaks (Suhrcke, Stuckler, Suk, Desai, Senek, McKee, and Rechel, 2011; Šumilo, Bormane, Asokliene, Vasilenko, Golovljova, Avsic-Zupanc, and Randolph, 2008).

Studies on epidemics and responses to them have argued that "acts of agreement" between key actors regarding the nature and definition of an epidemic are critical to clarifying courses of action such as policies, practices, and protocols (Poundstone, Strathdee, and Celentano, 2004; Pritchett, Thilmany, and Johnson, 2005; Pugliatti, Beghi, Forsgren, Ekman, and Sobocki, 2007). Consensus in identifying an outbreak helps define the roles of key protagonists, including international actors (in this case the WHO) and central and state government agencies (Armelagos, Brown, and Turner, 2005; Arokiasamy and Krishnan, 1994; Arora, 2001, 2005; Arredondo and Zúñiga, 2004). The WHO's interpretation of the plague outbreak must be framed within its efforts in the 1990s to explore a new global role for itself (Krieger, 2001a, b; Lemma, 1969; Liu, Maniadakis,

Gray, and Rayner, 2002; López, Torné, Franco, San-Martin, Viayna, Barrull, and Perulero, 2018). The effort to mobilize support for a new agenda among WHO advocates was drawn in part from challenges to its resources and role because of fund deficits and the competing roles of the United Nations Children's Fund (UNICEF) and World Bank (Amuna and Zotor, 2008; Aral, Holmes, Padian, and Cates, 1996; Arbabi, Nezami, Hooshyar, and Delavari, 2018). This is in addition to an emerging interest in forming new alignments and seeking support through private foundations and partnerships (Acemoglu and Johnson, 2007; Adda, 2016; Alloul, Sauriol, Kennedy, Laurier, Tessier, Novosel, and Contandriopoulos, 1998).

The World Health Organization's concerns regarding reemerging infections and global disease surveillance networks partially stemmed from concerns voiced among United States-based agencies (e.g., CDC and the Institute of Medicine) regarding the threat posed by new and reemerging infections to human security and social stability (St George, 1986; Steben and Duarte-Franco, 2007; Stehr-Green and Schantz, 1987; Stuckler, 2008; Stuckler and Siegel, 2011). This was particularly concerning in the new, interconnected geopolitical landscape of global health (Uusküla, Müürsepp, Kawai, Raag, Jürisson, and Pillsbury, 2013; Vanni, Karnon, Madan, White, Edmunds, Foss, and Legood, 2011). These infections, with their epicenters in Asia and Africa,38 were associated with HIV/AIDS and recent outbreaks such as monkeypox, hemorrhagic fevers, and drug-resistant tuberculosis (Perry and Randolph, 1999; Philipson, 2000; Philipson and Posner, 1996; Pongchaiyakul, Songpattanasilp, and Taechakraichana, 2008). It is also important to acknowledge the process through which human rights are curtailed in order to deal with the bigger threat of the epidemic (Weycker, Edelsberg, Oster, and Tino, 2005; Wu, Perrings, Kinzig, Collins, Minteer, and Daszak, 2017; Yach, Stuckler, and Brownell, 2006). In the case of COVID-19 governments have been able to curtail freedom of movement in ways that would have been unthinkable a few years ago (Chen, Li, Hsieh, Chang, Lee, Lee, and Ko, 2012; Conover, Pitt, Kessler, DuBow, and Sanborn, 1995; Crump, Murdoch, and Baker, 2001). Those who are interested in the political dynamics of disease epidemics question whether the so-called "social distancing dictates" are really a front for governments that are ravenous for power at all costs (Kim and Goldie, 2008; Klein, Laxminarayan, Smith, and Gilligan, 2007; Klepac, Laxminarayan, and Grenfell, 2011). In the next section, we explore the social dynamics of disease epidemics.

8.2. SOCIAL DYNAMICS OF DISEASE EPIDEMICS

The sociology of health and illness, alternatively the sociology of health and wellness (or simply health sociology), examines the interaction between society and health (Abegunde and Stanciole, 2008; Abramowitz, Lacau Saint Guily, Moyal-Barracco, Bergeron, Borne, Dahlab, and Bénard, 2018). The objective of this discipline is to see how social life affects morbidity and mortality rate, and vice versa (Jenkins, Baingana, Ahmad, McDaid, and Atun, 2011; Johnson, Alvarez-Pasquin, Bijl, Franco, Gaillat, Clara, and Weinke, 2015). This aspect of sociology differs from medical sociology in that this branch of sociology discusses health and illness in relation to social institutions such as family, employment, and school (Pal, Kerorsa, Marami, and Kandi, 2020; Paterson, Otte, Slingenbergh, Wint, and Rogers, 2000; Pearce and Merletti, 2006). The sociology of medicine limits its concern to the patient-practitioner relationship and the role of health professionals in society (Yi-Xin and Manderson, 2005; Zadoks, 2008; Zhan, Li, Wang, Sun, Geng, Xiong, and de Hoog, 2015; Zhang, Song, Cai, and Zhou, 2008). The sociology of health and illness covers sociological pathology (causes of disease and illness), reasons for seeking particular types of medical aid, and patient compliance or noncompliance with medical regimes (Bwire, Munier, Ouedraogo, Heyerdahl, Komakech, Kagirita, and Makumbi, 2017; Canali, Aragrande, Angheben, Capelli, Drigo, Gobbi, and Cassini, 2020). Figure 8.2 summarizes some of the sociological determinants of health experiences, including personal characteristics and the environment.

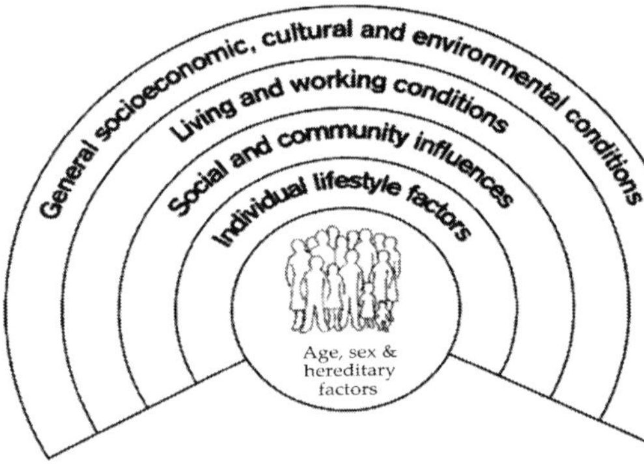

Figure 8.2. Sociological determinants of health experiences.

Source: Health Knowledge.

Health, or lack of health, was once merely attributed to biological or natural conditions (Buckley, 1984; Budke, Jiamin, Qian, and Torgerson, 2005; Bundy, Arámbulo III, and Grey, 1983; Buzby and Roberts, 2009). Sociologists have demonstrated that the spread of diseases is heavily influenced by the socioeconomic status of individuals, ethnic traditions or beliefs, and other cultural factors (Espinoza, Terashima, Herrera-Velit, and Marcos, 2010; Ezzati, Vander Hoorn, Lawes, Leach, James, Lopez, and Murray, 2005). Where medical research might gather statistics on a disease, a sociological perspective on an illness would provide insight on what external factors caused the demographics who contracted the disease to become ill (Bonds, Keenan, Rohani, and Sachs, 2010; Boni, Galvani, Wickelgren, and Malani, 2013; Bonovas and Nikolopoulos, 2012). This discipline requires a global approach of analysis because the influence of societal factors varies throughout the world (Ozmen, Kurşun, and Ozcelik, 2005; Paarlberg, Hillberg, Lee, and Mathews, 2008; Paisley, Vraa-Andersen, Dybkjaer, Møller, Christensen, Mousing, and Agger, 1993). This will be demonstrated through discussion of the major diseases of each continent (Casamassimo, Thikkurissy, Edelstein, and Maiorini, 2009; Castro, Wilson, and Bloom, 2017).

These diseases are sociologically examined and compared based on the traditional medicine, economics, religion, and culture that is specific to each region (Poundstone, Strathdee, and Celentano, 2004; Pritchett, Thilmany, and Johnson, 2005; Pugliatti, Beghi, Forsgren, Ekman, and Sobocki, 2007). HIV/AIDS serves as a common basis of comparison among regions (St George, 1986; Steben and Duarte-Franco, 2007; Stehr-Green and Schantz, 1987; Stuckler, 2008; Stuckler and Siegel, 2011). While it is extremely problematic in certain areas, in others it has affected a relatively small percentage of the population (Kim and Goldie, 2008; Klein, Laxminarayan, Smith, and Gilligan, 2007; Klepac, Laxminarayan, and Grenfell, 2011). Sociological factors can help to explain why these discrepancies exist (Bonds, Keenan, Rohani, and Sachs, 2010; Boni, Galvani, Wickelgren, and Malani, 2013; Bonovas and Nikolopoulos, 2012).

There are obvious differences in patterns of health and illness across societies, over time, and within particular society types (Oleś, Gudowska-Nowak, and Kleczkowski, 2012; Otte, Nugent, and McLeod, 2004; Ozawa, Portnoy, Getaneh, Clark, Knoll, Bishai, and Patwardhan, 2016). There has historically been a long-term decline in mortality within industrialized societies, and on average, life-expectancies are considerably higher in developed, rather than developing or undeveloped, societies (Armelagos,

Brown, and Turner, 2005; Arokiasamy and Krishnan, 1994; Arora, 2001, 2005; Arredondo and Zúñiga, 2004). Patterns of global change in health care systems make it more imperative than ever to research and comprehend the sociology of health and illness (Bwire, Munier, Ouedraogo, Heyerdahl, Komakech, Kagirita, and Makumbi, 2017; Canali, Aragrande, Angheben, Capelli, Drigo, Gobbi, and Cassini, 2020). Continuous changes in economy, therapy, technology, and insurance can affect the way individual communities view and respond to the medical care available (Borghol, Suderman, McArdle, Racine, Hallett, Pembrey, and Szyf, 2012; Brandes, 2008; Brown, Lipscomb, and Snyder, 2001). These rapid fluctuations cause the issue of health and illness within social life to be very dynamic in definition (Peckham, 2013; Perrings et al., 2002, 2014). Advancing information is vital because as patterns evolve, the study of the sociology of health and illness constantly needs to be updated (Amuna and Zotor, 2008; Aral, Holmes, Padian, and Cates, 1996; Arbabi, Nezami, Hooshyar, and Delavari, 2018).

Humans have long sought advice from those with knowledge or skill in healing (Acemoglu and Johnson, 2007; Adda, 2016; Alloul, Sauriol, Kennedy, Laurier, Tessier, Novosel, and Contandriopoulos, 1998). Paleopathology and other historical records, allow an examination of how ancient societies dealt with illness and outbreak (Eaton and Groopman, 2013; Eckelman, Sherman, and MacNeill, 2018; Egger, 2011; Elbe, 2007; Ernst and Hay, 1994). Rulers in Ancient Egypt sponsored physicians that were specialists in specific diseases (Espinoza, Terashima, Herrera-Velit, and Marcos, 2010; Ezzati, Vander Hoorn, Lawes, Leach, James, Lopez, and Murray, 2005). Imhotep was the first medical doctor known by name. An Egyptian who lived around 2650; B.C., he was an adviser to King Zoser at a time when Egyptians were making progress in medicine (Markos and Abdela, 2016; Martin and Shepherd, 2009; McGuinness, McGlynn, Johnson, MacIntyre, Batty, Burns, and McGinty, 2012). Among his contributions to medicine was a textbook on the treatment of wounds, broken bones, and even tumors (Suhrcke, Stuckler, Suk, Desai, Senek, McKee, and Rechel, 2011; Šumilo, Bormane, Asokliene, Vasilenko, Golovljova, Avsic-Zupanc, and Randolph, 2008). Stopping the spread of infectious disease was of utmost importance for maintaining a healthy society (Bergevoet, Van Schaik, Veling, Backus, and Franken, 2009; Binder, 1988; Bolos, Bacarea, and Marusteri, 2011). The outbreak of disease during the Peloponnesian War was recorded by Thucydides who survived the epidemic (Tapia, 2003; Torgerson and Dowling, 2001; Torgerson, Carmona, and Bonifacino, 2000; Uddin Khan, Atanasova, Krueger, Ramirez, and Gray, 2013). From his account, it is shown how factors outside the disease itself can affect society (Moné, Ibikounlé, Massougbodji, and Mouahid, 2010; Morand, 2004; Moro, Budke, Schantz, Vasquez, Santivanez, and Villavicencio, 2011). The Athenians were under siege and concentrated within the city. Major city centers were the hardest hit. This made the outbreak even more deadly and with probable food shortages the fate of Athens was inevitable (Uusküla, Müürsepp, Kawai, Raag, Jürisson, and Pillsbury, 2013; Vanni, Karnon, Madan, White, Edmunds, Foss, and Legood, 2011).

Ancient medical systems stressed the importance of reducing illness through divination and ritual (Raut, 2004; Rehm, Mathers, Popova, Thavorncharoensap, Teerawattananon, and Patra, 2009; Rich and Perry, 2011). Other codes of behavior and dietary protocols were widespread in the ancient world (Foxman, 2002; Garner, Whan, Gard, and Phillips, 2001; Gayle and Hill, 2001; Gottstein, Pozio, and Nöckler, 2009). During the Zhou Dynasty in China, doctors suggested exercise, meditation, and temperance to preserve one's health (Howe, Häsler, and Stärk, 2013; Howe et al., 2012). The Chinese closely link health with spiritual well-being (Weycker, Edelsberg, Oster, and Tino, 2005; Wu, Perrings, Kinzig, Collins, Minteer, and Daszak, 2017; Yach, Stuckler, and Brownell, 2006). Health regimes in ancient India focused on oral health as the best method for a healthy life (Daily, and Ehrlich, 1996; Deogaonkar, Hutubessy, Van Der Putten, Evers, and Jit, 2012; Dorn, 1992; Ducrotoy, Bertu, Ocholi, Gusi, Bryssinckx, Welburn, and Moriyon, 2014). The Talmudic code created rules for health which stressed ritual cleanliness, connected disease with certain animals and created diets (Chen, Li, Hsieh, Chang, Lee, Lee, and Ko, 2012; Conover, Pitt, Kessler, DuBow, and Sanborn, 1995; Crump, Murdoch, and Baker, 2001). Other examples include the Mosaic Code and Roman baths and aqueducts (Arredondo and Zúñiga, 2006; Backer, van Roermund, Fischer, van Asseldonk, and Bergevoet, 2015; Bartsch, Hotez, Hertenstein, Diemert, Zapf, Bottazzi, and Lee, 2016).

Those that were most concerned with health, sanitation, and illness in the ancient world were those in the elite class (Rogers, Carolin, Vaught, and Compton, 2011; Ronohardjo and Rastiko, 1982; Sachs, 2001; Sachs and Malaney, 2002). Good health was thought to reduce the risk of spiritual defilement and therefore enhanced the social status of the ruling class who saw themselves as the beacon of civilization (Yi-Xin and Manderson, 2005; Zadoks, 2008; Zhan, Li, Wang, Sun, Geng, Xiong, and de Hoog, 2015; Zhang, Song, Cai, and Zhou, 2008). During the late Roman Period, sanitation for the lower classes was a concern for the leisured class (Perry and Randolph,

1999; Philipson, 2000; Philipson and Posner, 1996; Pongchaiyakul, Songpattanasilp, and Taechakraichana, 2008). Those that had the means would donate to charities that focused on the health of non-elites (Abegunde and Stanciole, 2008; Abramowitz, Lacau Saint Guily, Moyal-Barracco, Bergeron, Borne, Dahlab, and Bénard, 2018). After the decline of the Roman Empire, physicians, and concern with public health disappeared except in the largest cities (Fenichel, 2013; Fenichel et al., 2011; Fogel, 1994). Health and public doctors remained in the Byzantine Empire (Saleha, 1991; Sibert, Rigaud, Delavierre, and Labat, 2010; Skrepnek and Skrepnek, 2004; Sloane, 2009; Sockett, 1993). Focusing on preventing the spread of diseases such as small pox lead to a smaller mortality rate in much of the western world (Bausch and Schwarz, 2014; Bausch et al., 2001; Benner, Carabin, Sánchez-Serrano, Budke, and Carmena, 2010). Other factors that allowed the modern rise in population include: better nutrition and environmental reforms (Hart and Halden, 2020; Häsler, Howe, and Stärk, 2011; Henschke, Kamper, and Maher, 2015; Hochberg, 1992).

The present-day sense of health being a public concern for the state began in the Middle Ages (Ozmen, Kurşun, and Ozcelik, 2005; Paarlberg, Hillberg, Lee, and Mathews, 2008; Paisley, Vraa-Andersen, Dybkjaer, Møller, Christensen, Mousing, and Agger, 1993). A few state interventions include maintaining clean towns, enforcing quarantines during epidemics and supervising sewer systems (Buckley, 1984; Budke, Jiamin, Qian, and Torgerson, 2005; Bundy, Arámbulo III, and Grey, 1983; Buzby and Roberts, 2009). Private corporations also played a role in public health (Pal, Kerorsa, Marami, and Kandi, 2020; Paterson, Otte, Slingenbergh, Wint, and Rogers, 2000; Pearce and Merletti, 2006). The funding for research and the institutions for them to work were funded by governments and private firms (Narrod, Zinsstag, and Tiongco, 2012; Nascimento and de Oliveira, 2014; O'Brien, Lahue, Caro, and Davidson, 2007). Epidemics were the cause of most government interventions (Krieger, 2001a, b; Lemma, 1969; Liu, Maniadakis, Gray, and Rayner, 2002; López, Torné, Franco, San-Martin, Viayna, Barrull, and Perulero, 2018). The early goal of public health was reactionary, whereas the modern goal is to prevent disease before it becomes a problem (Jenkins, Baingana, Ahmad, McDaid, and Atun, 2011; Johnson, Alvarez-Pasquin, Bijl, Franco, Gaillat, Clara, and Weinke, 2015). Despite the overall improvement of world health, there still has not been any decrease in the health gap between the affluent and the impoverished (Purevdawa, Moon, Baigalmaa, Davaajav, Smith, and Vermund, 1997; Ramesh, Malla, Raju, Sehgal, Ganguly, Mahajan, and Dilawari, 1990).

Today, society is more likely to blame health issues on the individual rather than society as a whole (Jenkins, Baingana, Ahmad, McDaid, and Atun, 2011; Johnson, Alvarez-Pasquin, Bijl, Franco, Gaillat, Clara, and Weinke, 2015). This was the prevailing view in the late 20th century (Krieger, 2001a, b; Lemma, 1969; Liu, Maniadakis, Gray, and Rayner, 2002; López, Torné, Franco, San-Martin, Viayna, Barrull, and Perulero, 2018). In the 1980s, the Black Report, published in the United Kingdom, went against this view and argued that the true root of the problem was material deprivation (Narrod, Zinsstag, and Tiongco, 2012; Nascimento and de Oliveira, 2014; O'Brien, Lahue, Caro, and Davidson, 2007). This report proposed a comprehensive anti-poverty strategy to address these issues (Pal, Kerorsa, Marami, and Kandi, 2020; Paterson, Otte, Slingenbergh, Wint, and Rogers, 2000; Pearce and Merletti, 2006). Since this did not parallel the views of the Conservative government, it did not go into action immediately (Buckley, 1984; Budke, Jiamin, Qian, and Torgerson, 2005; Bundy, Arámbulo III, and Grey, 1983; Buzby and Roberts, 2009).

The Conservative government was criticized by the Labor Party for not implementing the suggestions that the Black Report listed (Ozmen, Kurşun, and Ozcelik, 2005; Paarlberg, Hillberg, Lee, and Mathews, 2008; Paisley, Vraa-Andersen, Dybkjaer, Møller, Christensen, Mousing, and Agger, 1993). This criticism gave the Black Report the exposure it needed and its arguments were considered a valid explanation for health inequality (Hart and Halden, 2020; Häsler, Howe, and Stärk, 2011; Henschke, Kamper, and Maher, 2015; Hochberg, 1992). There is also a debate over whether poverty causes ill-health or if ill-health causes poverty (Bausch and Schwarz, 2014; Bausch et al., 2001; Benner, Carabin, Sánchez-Serrano, Budke, and Carmena, 2010). Arguments by the National Health Service gave considerable emphasis to poverty and lack of access to health care (Saleha, 1991; Sibert, Rigaud, Delavierre, and Labat, 2010; Skrepnek and Skrepnek, 2004; Sloane, 2009; Sockett, 1993). It has also been found that heredity has more of a bearing on health than social environment, but research has also proved that there is indeed a positive correlation between socioeconomic inequalities and illness (Fenichel, 2013; Fenichel et al., 2011; Fogel, 1994). More recently, sociological studies following a life course perspective in health emphasized the limitations of the view linking health outcomes on individual agency only (Abegunde and Stanciole, 2008; Abramowitz, Lacau Saint Guily, Moyal-Barracco, Bergeron, Borne, Dahlab, and Bénard, 2018).

The sociology of health and illness examines three areas including the conceptualization, the study of measurement and social distribution, and the justification of patterns in health and illness (Yi-Xin and Manderson, 2005; Zadoks, 2008; Zhan, Li, Wang, Sun, Geng, Xiong, and de Hoog, 2015; Zhang, Song, Cai, and Zhou, 2008). By looking at these things, researchers can look at different diseases through a sociological lens. The prevalence and response to different diseases varies by culture (Rogers, Carolin, Vaught, and Compton, 2011; Ronohardjo and Rastiko, 1982; Sachs, 2001; Sachs and Malaney, 2002). By analyzing bad health, researchers can see if health affects different social regulations or controls (Arredondo and Zúñiga, 2006; Backer, van Roermund, Fischer, van Asseldonk, and Bergevoet, 2015; Bartsch, Hotez, Hertenstein, Diemert, Zapf, Bottazzi, and Lee, 2016). When measuring the distribution of health and illness, it is useful to look at official statistics and community surveys (Chen, Li, Hsieh, Chang, Lee, Lee, and Ko, 2012; Conover, Pitt, Kessler, DuBow, and Sanborn, 1995; Crump, Murdoch, and Baker, 2001). Official statistics make it possible to look at people who have been treated (Daily, and Ehrlich, 1996; Deogaonkar, Hutubessy, Van Der Putten, Evers, and Jit, 2012; Dorn, 1992; Ducrotoy, Bertu, Ocholi, Gusi, Bryssinckx, Welburn, and Moriyon, 2014). It shows that they are both willing and able to use health services (Weycker, Edelsberg, Oster, and Tino, 2005; Wu, Perrings, Kinzig, Collins, Minteer, and Daszak, 2017; Yach, Stuckler, and Brownell, 2006). It also sheds light on the infected person's view of their illness (Howe, Häsler, and Stärk, 2013; Howe et al., 2012). On the other hand, community surveys look at people's rating of their health (Foxman, 2002; Garner, Whan, Gard, and Phillips, 2001; Gayle and Hill, 2001; Gottstein, Pozio, and Nöckler, 2009). Then looking at the relation of clinically defined illness and self-reports and find that there is often a discrepancy (Raut, 2004; Rehm, Mathers, Popova, Thavorncharoensap, Teerawattananon, and Patra, 2009; Rich and Perry, 2011).

A great deal of the time, mortality statistics take the place of the morbidity statistics because in many developed societies where people typically die from degenerative conditions, the age in which they die sheds lighter on their life-time health (Uusküla, Müürsepp, Kawai, Raag, Jürisson, and Pillsbury, 2013; Vanni, Karnon, Madan, White, Edmunds, Foss, and Legood, 2011). This produces many limitations when looking at the pattern of sickness, but sociologists try to look at various data to analyze the distribution better (Moné, Ibikounlé, Massougbodji, and Mouahid, 2010; Morand, 2004; Moro, Budke, Schantz, Vasquez, Santivanez, and Villavicencio, 2011). Normally, developing societies have lower life expectancies in comparison to developed countries (Tapia, 2003; Torgerson and Dowling, 2001; Torgerson, Carmona, and Bonifacino, 2000; Uddin Khan, Atanasova, Krueger, Ramirez, and

Gray, 2013). They have also found correlations between mortality and sex and age (Bergevoet, Van Schaik, Veling, Backus, and Franken, 2009; Binder, 1988; Bolos, Bacarea, and Marusteri, 2011). Very young and old people are more susceptible to sickness and death (Suhrcke, Stuckler, Suk, Desai, Senek, McKee, and Rechel, 2011; Šumilo, Bormane, Asokliene, Vasilenko, Golovljova, Avsic-Zupanc, and Randolph, 2008). On average, women typically live longer than men, although women are more likely to have bad health (Markos and Abdela, 2016; Martin and Shepherd, 2009; McGuinness, McGlynn, Johnson, MacIntyre, Batty, Burns, and McGinty, 2012).

Disparities in health were also found between people in different social classes and ethnicities within the same society (Espinoza, Terashima, Herrera-Velit, and Marcos, 2010; Ezzati, Vander Hoorn, Lawes, Leach, James, Lopez, and Murray, 2005). This holds true despite the fact that the medical profession places more importance in "health-related behaviors" such as alcohol consumption, smoking, diet, and exercise (Eaton and Groopman, 2013; Eckelman, Sherman, and MacNeill, 2018; Egger, 2011; Elbe, 2007; Ernst and Hay, 1994). There is a great deal of data supporting the conclusion that these behaviors affect health more significantly than other factors (Acemoglu and Johnson, 2007; Adda, 2016; Alloul, Sauriol, Kennedy, Laurier, Tessier, Novosel, and Contandriopoulos, 1998). Sociologists are of the view that it is more helpful to look at health and illness through a broad lens. Sociologists agree that alcohol consumption, smoking, diet, and exercise are important issues (Amuna and Zotor, 2008; Aral, Holmes, Padian, and Cates, 1996; Arbabi, Nezami, Hooshyar, and Delavari, 2018). However, they also see the importance of analyzing the cultural factors that affect these patterns. Sociologists also look at the effects that the productive process has on health and illness (Peckham, 2013; Perrings et al., 2002, 2014). While also looking at things such as industrial pollution, environmental pollution, accidents at work, and stress-related diseases (Borghol, Suderman, McArdle, Racine, Hallett, Pembrey, and Szyf, 2012; Brandes, 2008; Brown, Lipscomb, and Snyder, 2001).

Social factors play a significant role in developing health and illness (Bwire, Munier, Ouedraogo, Heyerdahl, Komakech, Kagirita, and Makumbi, 2017; Canali, Aragrande, Angheben, Capelli, Drigo, Gobbi, and Cassini, 2020). Studies of epidemiology show that autonomy and control in the workplace are vital factors in the etiology of heart disease (Armelagos, Brown, and Turner, 2005; Arokiasamy and Krishnan, 1994; Arora, 2001, 2005; Arredondo and Zúñiga, 2004). One cause is an effort-reward imbalance. Decreasing career advancement opportunities and major imbalances in control over work have been coupled with various negative health costs (Oleś, Gudowska-Nowak, and Kleczkowski, 2012; Otte, Nugent, and McLeod, 2004; Ozawa, Portnoy, Getaneh, Clark, Knoll, Bishai, and Patwardhan, 2016). Various studies have shown that pension rights may shed light on mortality differences between retired men and women of different socioeconomic statuses (Bonds, Keenan, Rohani, and Sachs, 2010; Boni, Galvani, Wickelgren, and Malani, 2013; Bonovas and Nikolopoulos, 2012). These studies show that there are outside factors that influence health and illness (Kim and Goldie, 2008; Klein, Laxminarayan, Smith, and Gilligan, 2007; Klepac, Laxminarayan, and Grenfell, 2011). In the next section, we consider the economic responses to disease epidemicsDisease epidemics.

8.3. ECONOMIC RESPONSES TO DISEASE EPIDEMICS

Despite the crucial nature of the subject, only a few reliable studies have been produced for this field of social medicine so far (St George, 1986; Steben and Duarte-Franco, 2007; Stehr-Green and Schantz, 1987; Stuckler, 2008; Stuckler and Siegel, 2011). Most studies rely on historical case studies so as to calibrate the parameters of the respective models (Poundstone, Strathdee, and Celentano, 2004; Pritchett, Thilmany, and Johnson, 2005; Pugliatti, Beghi, Forsgren, Ekman, and Sobocki, 2007). Whereas macroeconomic models are primarily aimed at quantifying the effects of rapidly spreading infectious diseases, actuarial mathematics links the expected effects to probabilities (Casamassimo, Thikkurissy, Edelstein, and Maiorini, 2009; Castro, Wilson, and Bloom, 2017). The idea is to forecast the probability of pandemics and their socio-economic costs. The various studies and their models forecast relatively limited economic effects (Yi-Xin and Manderson, 2005; Zadoks, 2008; Zhan, Li, Wang, Sun, Geng, Xiong, and de Hoog, 2015; Zhang, Song, Cai, and Zhou, 2008). On average, experts envisage a decline of global economic output (as measured by GDP) of 0.6% or USD 500 bn (Weycker, Edelsberg, Oster, and Tino, 2005; Wu, Perrings, Kinzig, Collins, Minteer, and Daszak, 2017; Yach, Stuckler, and Brownell, 2006). At the same time, the consensus expects a V-shaped recovery of the economy in the coming 3 to 12 months (Uusküla, Müürsepp, Kawai, Raag, Jürisson, and Pillsbury, 2013; Vanni, Karnon, Madan, White, Edmunds, Foss, and Legood, 2011). That being said, significant regional differences are likely, especially in terms of the effects on the GDP of the first world when compared to developing economies (Tapia, 2003; Torgerson and Dowling, 2001; Torgerson, Carmona, and Bonifacino, 2000; Uddin Khan, Atanasova, Krueger, Ramirez, and Gray, 2013). Figure 8.3 highlights the human and social costs of disease pandemics over the years.

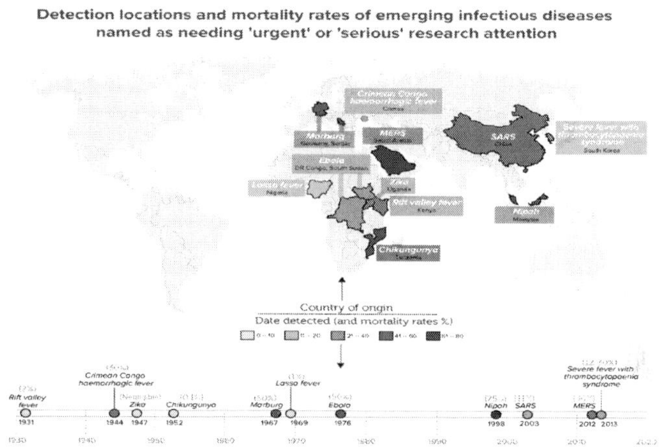

Figure 8.3. Human and economic costs of disease pandemics.

Source: World Economic Forum.

The most negative estimate of a study with regard to an assumed outbreak of Ebola in Sierra Leone suggested a slump in GDP of 16% in this economy (Suhrcke, Stuckler, Suk, Desai, Senek, McKee, and Rechel, 2011; Šumilo, Bormane, Asokliene, Vasilenko, Golovljova, Avsic-Zupanc, and Randolph, 2008). This was due to the, relatively to industrialized states, deficient healthcare, the generally worse supply situation within the population, and the high population density in conjunction with a lack of hygiene (St George, 1986; Steben and Duarte-Franco, 2007; Stehr-Green and Schantz, 1987; Stuckler, 2008; Stuckler and Siegel, 2011). In a 2013 model, the World Bank set the probability of a global pandemic at 1% to 3%. This is very low, but in the event of a high rate of infection (like for the Spanish flu), the costs for the global economy could amount to as much as USD 3,000 bn (Saleha, 1991; Sibert, Rigaud, Delavierre, and Labat, 2010; Skrepnek and Skrepnek, 2004; Sloane, 2009; Sockett, 1993). In view of this volume, the World Bank warns that the community of states has set insufficient preventive measures. According to its model, USD 3.7 bn would have to be invested annually in preventive measures (especially in developing countries) for the cost caused by infectious diseases to fall by USD 37 bn. Generally speaking, the economic cost is biggest in those sectors where personal client contact takes place and where consumption cannot be suspended (Rogers, Carolin, Vaught, and Compton, 2011; Ronohardjo and Rastiko, 1982; Sachs, 2001; Sachs and Malaney, 2002). This includes numerous segments of the service sector, especially tourism and the leisure industry (Raut, 2004; Rehm, Mathers, Popova, Thavorncharoensap, Teerawattananon, and Patra, 2009; Rich and Perry, 2011). Companies with complex and global supply chains that would be disrupted by the fight against a pandemic would also be particularly hard hit (Purevdawa, Moon, Baigalmaa, Davaajav, Smith, and Vermund, 1997; Ramesh, Malla, Raju, Sehgal, Ganguly, Mahajan, and Dilawari, 1990). In terms of countries, those economies would be worst affected that strongly depended on the input factor labor (Poundstone, Strathdee, and Celentano, 2004; Pritchett, Thilmany, and Johnson, 2005; Pugliatti, Beghi, Forsgren, Ekman, and Sobocki, 2007). This means that developing countries would feel the costs of an epidemic or pandemic more severely than developed countries, given that their economy is less significantly automatized and digitized (Perry and Randolph, 1999; Philipson, 2000; Philipson and Posner, 1996; Pongchaiyakul, Songpattanasilp, and Taechakraichana, 2008).

The degree of interconnectedness of regions is another important influencing factor for the spreading of an infectious disease and costs associated with it (Peckham, 2013; Perrings et al., 2002, 2014). For example, a virus will spread faster in open economies such as Europe than, say, in the Middle East, where the individual countries are more isolated from each other (Pal, Kerorsa, Marami, and Kandi, 2020; Paterson, Otte, Slingenbergh, Wint, and Rogers, 2000; Pearce and Merletti, 2006). An important element with regard to the costs generated by pandemics is human behavior (Ozmen, Kurşun, and Ozcelik, 2005; Paarlberg, Hillberg, Lee, and Mathews, 2008; Paisley, Vraa-Andersen, Dybkjaer, Møller, Christensen, Mousing, and Agger, 1993). Fear of contagion can be both detrimental to containment and produce immediate negative economic effects (Oleś, Gudowska-Nowak, and Kleczkowski, 2012; Otte, Nugent, and McLeod, 2004; Ozawa, Portnoy, Getaneh, Clark, Knoll, Bishai, and Patwardhan, 2016). This starts at the sociology of a quarantine situation, which people will try to escape in order to avoid possible contagion and thus carry the virus with them (Narrod, Zinsstag, and Tiongco, 2012; Nascimento and de Oliveira, 2014; O'Brien, Lahue, Caro, and Davidson, 2007).

Existing studies suggest that many people resort to self-quarantine so as to avoid contracting a virus (Moné, Ibikounlé, Massougbodji, and Mouahid,

2010; Morand, 2004; Moro, Budke, Schantz, Vasquez, Santivanez, and Villavicencio, 2011). This self-quarantine includes the avoidance of places that are associated with a heightened risk of contagion (e.g., events, restaurants, cinemas, traveling, etc.), which has a negative effect on consumption (Markos and Abdela, 2016; Martin and Shepherd, 2009; McGuinness, McGlynn, Johnson, MacIntyre, Batty, Burns, and McGinty, 2012). As previous pandemics have shown, in particularly affected areas people also stay away from work so as to avoid infection (Krieger, 2001a, b; Lemma, 1969; Liu, Maniadakis, Gray, and Rayner, 2002; López, Torné, Franco, San-Martin, Viayna, Barrull, and Perulero, 2018). According to research, such forms of voluntarily taken protective measures account for about 60% of the knock-on costs of a pandemic (Kim and Goldie, 2008; Klein, Laxminarayan, Smith, and Gilligan, 2007; Klepac, Laxminarayan, and Grenfell, 2011). The most significant issue is the global increase in traffic over recent decades (Jenkins, Baingana, Ahmad, McDaid, and Atun, 2011; Johnson, Alvarez-Pasquin, Bijl, Franco, Gaillat, Clara, and Weinke, 2015). This includes both the transportation of cargo and people traveling (Howe, Häsler, and Stärk, 2013; Howe et al., 2012). Additionally, supply chains have become significantly more globalized in recent years (Hart and Halden, 2020; Häsler, Howe, and Stärk, 2011; Henschke, Kamper, and Maher, 2015; Hochberg, 1992). All of that has drastically increased the level of integration in the global economy (Foxman, 2002; Garner, Whan, Gard, and Phillips, 2001; Gayle and Hill, 2001; Gottstein, Pozio, and Nöckler, 2009).

After all, the economic environment is more challenging than many a previous pandemic (Fenichel, 2013; Fenichel et al., 2011; Fogel, 1994). After several years of strong growth, economic growth is currently in a phase of slowdown (Espinoza, Terashima, Herrera-Velit, and Marcos, 2010; Ezzati, Vander Hoorn, Lawes, Leach, James, Lopez, and Murray, 2005). At the same time, the share of China and South East Asia in total global economic output has increased substantially in the recent 10 years (Eaton and Groopman, 2013; Eckelman, Sherman, and MacNeill, 2018; Egger, 2011; Elbe, 2007; Ernst and Hay, 1994). A pandemic, not the least one that originated in China, could therefore come with a stronger effect on the global economy in such an environment than previous pandemics (Daily, and Ehrlich, 1996; Deogaonkar, Hutubessy, Van Der Putten, Evers, and Jit, 2012; Dorn, 1992; Ducrotoy, Bertu, Ocholi, Gusi, Bryssinckx, Welburn, and Moriyon, 2014). In addition, the central banks have little room to thwart possible negative consequences effectively amid the current phase of low interest rates (Chen, Li, Hsieh, Chang, Lee, Lee, and Ko, 2012; Conover, Pitt, Kessler, DuBow, and Sanborn, 1995; Crump, Murdoch, and Baker, 2001). A study from 2006 for example, makes the recommendation to the ECB to cut its key lending rates by 100 bps as first countermeasure (Casamassimo, Thikkurissy, Edelstein, and Maiorini, 2009; Castro, Wilson, and Bloom, 2017). Such an intervention would not really be possible nowadays (Bwire, Munier, Ouedraogo, Heyerdahl, Komakech, Kagirita, and Makumbi, 2017; Canali, Aragrande, Angheben, Capelli, Drigo, Gobbi, and Cassini, 2020). Social media, having gained a strong foothold in our society in the recent 10 years, are another important aspect (Buckley, 1984; Budke, Jiamin, Qian, and Torgerson, 2005; Bundy, Arámbulo III, and Grey, 1983; Buzby and Roberts, 2009). They can amplify the panic and thus further push up the costs of a pandemic (Borghol, Suderman, McArdle, Racine, Hallett, Pembrey, and Szyf, 2012; Brandes, 2008; Brown, Lipscomb, and Snyder, 2001). While the odd younger study does point out this effect, it has not entered the models yet (Bonds, Keenan, Rohani, and Sachs, 2010; Boni, Galvani, Wickelgren, and Malani, 2013; Bonovas and Nikolopoulos, 2012).

While no final conclusions have been reached about the rampant coronavirus due to the early stages we are in, the progress so far allows for a few initial learning points (Bergevoet, Van Schaik, Veling, Backus, and Franken, 2009; Binder, 1988; Bolos, Bacarea, and Marusteri, 2011). The transmission rate of the coronavirus seems to be equal to that of a cold or an aggressive form of influenza (Bausch and Schwarz, 2014; Bausch et al., 2001; Benner, Carabin, Sánchez-Serrano, Budke, and Carmena, 2010). Here, one infected person passes on the virus to two other people (Arredondo and Zúñiga, 2006; Backer, van Roermund, Fischer, van Asseldonk, and Bergevoet, 2015; Bartsch, Hotez, Hertenstein, Diemert, Zapf, Bottazzi, and Lee, 2016). In terms of the mortality rate, the COVID-19 virus ranks slightly higher than the common influenza virus, but clearly below the SARS virus (Armelagos, Brown, and Turner, 2005; Arokiasamy and Krishnan, 1994; Arora, 2001, 2005; Arredondo and Zúñiga, 2004). Moreover, the demographic groups of people above 70 and above 80 years old seem to be affected at disproportionately high rates by a severe course of the disease. At the same time, the age group of employable people (especially 20 to 60) shows a milder development of the disease.

COVID-19 is not only a global pandemic and public health crisis; it has also severely affected the global economy and financial markets. Significant reductions in income, a rise in unemployment, and disruptions in the transportation, service, and manufacturing industries are among the consequences of the disease mitigation measures that have been implemented in many countries (Amuna and Zotor, 2008; Aral, Holmes, Padian, and Cates, 1996; Arbabi, Nezami, Hooshyar, and Delavari, 2018). It has become clear that most governments in the world underestimated the risks of rapid COVID-19 spread and were mostly reactive in their crisis response. As disease outbreaks are not likely to disappear in the near future, proactive international actions are required to not only save lives but also protect economic prosperity (Acemoglu and Johnson, 2007; Adda, 2016; Alloul, Sauriol, Kennedy, Laurier, Tessier, Novosel, and Contandriopoulos, 1998).

The WHO characterized COVID-19 as a pandemic. This was based on existing statistics showing that over 3 million cases and 207,973 deaths had occurred in 213 countries and territories. The infection has not only become a public health crisis but has also affected the global economy. Significant economic impact has already occurred across the globe due to reduced productivity, loss of life, business closures, trade disruption, and decimation of the tourism industry. COVID-19 may be that a "wake-up" call for global leaders to intensify cooperation on epidemic preparedness and provide the necessary financing for international collective action (Abegunde and Stanciole, 2008; Abramowitz, Lacau Saint Guily, Moyal-Barracco, Bergeron, Borne, Dahlab, and Bénard, 2018). There has been ample information on the expected economic and health costs of infectious disease outbreaks, but the world has failed to adequately invest in preventive and preparedness measures to mitigate the risks of large epidemics (Ozmen, Kurşun, and Ozcelik, 2005; Paarlberg, Hillberg, Lee, and Mathews, 2008; Paisley, Vraa-Andersen, Dybkjaer, Møller, Christensen, Mousing, and Agger, 1993).

With globalization, urbanization, and environmental change, infectious disease outbreaks and epidemics have become global threats requiring a collective response (Bonds, Keenan, Rohani, and Sachs, 2010; Boni, Galvani, Wickelgren, and Malani, 2013; Bonovas and Nikolopoulos, 2012). Although the majority of developed countries, predominantly European and North American, have strong real-time surveillance and health systems to manage infectious disease spread, improvements in public health capacity in low-income and high-risk countries (Espinoza, Terashima, Herrera-Velit, and Marcos, 2010; Ezzati, Vander Hoorn, Lawes, Leach, James, Lopez, and Murray, 2005). This includes human and animal surveillance, workforce preparedness, and strengthening laboratory resources (Buckley, 1984; Budke, Jiamin, Qian, and Torgerson, 2005; Bundy, Arámbulo III, and

Grey, 1983; Buzby and Roberts, 2009). Such measures need to be supported by using national resources supplemented with international donor funding (Bwire, Munier, Ouedraogo, Heyerdahl, Komakech, Kagirita, and Makumbi, 2017; Canali, Aragrande, Angheben, Capelli, Drigo, Gobbi, and Cassini, 2020). International collective action among governments, non-government organizations, and private companies has been advocated in building and financing technological platforms to accelerate the research on and development response to new pathogens with epidemic potential (Yi-Xin and Manderson, 2005; Zadoks, 2008; Zhan, Li, Wang, Sun, Geng, Xiong, and de Hoog, 2015; Zhang, Song, Cai, and Zhou, 2008).

In the case of COVID-19, such cooperation is critical, especially for the development and production of a vaccine (Pal, Kerorsa, Marami, and Kandi, 2020; Paterson, Otte, Slingenbergh, Wint, and Rogers, 2000; Pearce and Merletti, 2006). The Coalition for Epidemic Preparedness Innovations (CEPI), a global partnership launched in 2017, has tracked global efforts in COVID-19 vaccine development activity and is advocating for strong international cooperation to ensure that vaccine, when developed, will be manufactured in sufficient quantities and that equitable access will be provided to all nations regardless of ability to pay. Furthermore, affected countries may benefit from exchanging technological innovations in contact tracing, such as health quick response (QR) codes, to manage the outbreak more effectively (Jenkins, Baingana, Ahmad, McDaid, and Atun, 2011; Johnson, Alvarez-Pasquin, Bijl, Franco, Gaillat, Clara, and Weinke, 2015). However, there are important privacy implications that need to be considered (Abegunde and Stanciole, 2008; Abramowitz, Lacau Saint Guily, Moyal-Barracco, Bergeron, Borne, Dahlab, and Bénard, 2018). In the case of COVID-19, the collective response and adoption of preventive measures to stop the global spread were implemented too late, after COVID-19 had already penetrated other regions through international travel (Kim and Goldie, 2008; Klein, Laxminarayan, Smith, and Gilligan, 2007; Klepac, Laxminarayan, and Grenfell, 2011).

In addition to marked health inequalities, especially in countries without universal healthcare coverage, the economic impact of the COVID-19 pandemic will be heterogeneous across the country's income distribution (Chen, Li, Hsieh, Chang, Lee, Lee, and Ko, 2012; Conover, Pitt, Kessler, DuBow, and Sanborn, 1995; Crump, Murdoch, and Baker, 2001). For example, office workers are more likely to transition to flexible working arrangements during the restrictions, while many industrial, tourism, retail, and transport workers will suffer a significant reduction in work due to community restrictions and low demand for their goods and services (Weycker, Edelsberg, Oster, and Tino, 2005; Wu, Perrings, Kinzig, Collins, Minteer, and Daszak, 2017; Yach, Stuckler, and Brownell, 2006). Global financial markets have been heavily impacted by the effects of COVID-19 spread. As the numbers of cases started to increase globally, mainly through the US, Italy, Spain, Germany, France, Iran, and South Korea, the world financial and oil markets significantly declined.

CHAPTER 8 SUMMARY

This final chapter has shown that disease pandemics such as the recent COVID-19 outbreak have the capability of impacting on the political, economic, and social aspects of a community. The political response is about containment and control. Meanwhile, the economy has to deal with the changes in the workforce or even the ability of the populace to participate in economic activity. The social impact is main about the various responses from the community in terms of understanding and managing the epidemic. Overall, this chapter has shown that disease epidemicsDisease epidemics have an impact that goes beyond the illness and deaths that they cause.

Chapter 9

Concluding Remarks

This book was conceived as a pertinent commentary on the impact of disease epidemicsDisease epidemics on the economy. At a time when the world is in the midst of the COVID-19 crisis, the insights that are provided in this book are particularly relevant. The take-home message is really about the complexity of these disease epidemicsDisease epidemics. Typically, we are used to counting the cost of disease epidemicsDisease epidemics in terms of infection rates and fatalities. However, this book has shown that there is a lot more to disease epidemicsDisease epidemics than these two factors. The unique experiences of the communities that have been through these epidemics are instructive. This is because they can be strategically deployed to prevent and control further epidemics. I hope you have enjoyed reading the book and will explore the other items in the series.

Bibliography

1. Abegunde, D. O., & Stanciole, A. E., (2008). The economic impact of chronic diseases: How do households respond to shocks? Evidence from Russia. *Social Science and Medicine, 66*(11), 2296–2307.
2. Abramowitz, L., Lacau, S. G. J., Moyal-Barracco, M., Bergeron, C., Borne, H., Dahlab, A., & Bénard, S., (2018). Epidemiological and economic burden of potentially HPV-related cancers in France. *PloS One, 13*(9), e0202564.
3. Acemoglu, D., & Johnson, S., (2007). Disease and development: The effect of life expectancy on economic growth. *Journal of Political Economy, 115*(6), 925–985.
4. Adda, J., (2016). Economic activity and the spread of viral diseases: Evidence from high frequency data. *The Quarterly Journal of Economics, 131*(2), 891–941.
5. Alloul, K., Sauriol, L., Kennedy, W., Laurier, C., Tessier, G., Novosel, S., & Contandriopoulos, A., (1998). Alzheimer's disease: A review of the disease, its epidemiology and economic impact. *Archives of Gerontology and Geriatrics, 27*(3), 189–221.
6. Amuna, P., & Zotor, F. B., (2008). Epidemiological and nutrition transition in developing countries: Impact on human health and development: The epidemiological and nutrition transition in developing countries: Evolving trends and their impact in public health

and human development. *Proceedings of the Nutrition Society, 67*(1), 82–90.

7. Aral, S. O., Holmes, K. K., Padian, N. S., & Cates, W., (1996). Overview: Individual and population approaches to the epidemiology and prevention of sexually transmitted diseases and human immunodeficiency virus infection. *The Journal of Infectious Diseases, 174*, S127–S133.
8. Arbabi, M., Nezami, E., Hooshyar, H., & Delavari, M., (2018). Epidemiology and economic loss of fasciolosis and dicrocoeliasis in Arak, Iran. *Veterinary World, 11*(12), 1648.
9. Armelagos, G. J., Brown, P. J., & Turner, B., (2005). Evolutionary, historical and political-economic perspectives on health and disease. *Social Science and Medicine, 61*(4), 755–765.
10. Arokiasamy, J. T., & Krishnan, R., (1994). Some epidemiological aspects and economic costs of injuries in Malaysia. *Asia Pacific Journal of Public Health, 7*(1), 16–20.
11. Arora, S., (2001). Health, human productivity, and long-term economic growth. *The Journal of Economic History, 61*(3), 699–749.
12. Arora, S., (2005). *On Epidemiologic and Economic Transitions: A Historical View*., in Health and Economic Growth: Findings and Policy Implications, edited by G. Lopez Casasnovas, B. Rivera and L. Currais, MIT Press, Cambridge, MA, 197 – 238.
13. Arredondo, A., & Zúñiga, A., (2004). Economic consequences of epidemiological changes in diabetes in middle-income countries: The Mexican case. *Diabetes Care, 27*(1), 104–109.
14. Arredondo, A., & Zúñiga, A., (2006). Epidemiologic changes and economic burden of hypertension in Latin America: Evidence from Mexico. *American Journal of Hypertension, 19*(6), 553–559.
15. Backer, J. A., Van, R. H. J. W., Fischer, E. A. J., Van, A. M. A. P. M., & Bergevoet, R. H. M., (2015). Controlling highly pathogenic avian influenza outbreaks: An epidemiological and economic model analysis. *Preventive Veterinary Medicine, 121*(1, 2), 142–150.
16. Bartsch, S. M., Hotez, P. J., Hertenstein, D. L., Diemert, D. J., Zapf, K. M., Bottazzi, M. E., & Lee, B. Y., (2016). Modeling the economic and epidemiologic impact of hookworm vaccine and mass drug administration (MDA) in Brazil, a high transmission setting. *Vaccine, 34*(19), 2197–2206.

17. Bausch, D. G., & Schwarz, L., (2014). Outbreak of Ebola virus disease in Guinea: Where ecology meets economy. *PLoS Negl. Trop. Dis., 8*(7), e3056.

18. Bausch, D. G., Demby, A. H., Coulibaly, M., Kanu, J., Goba, A., Bah, A., & Baldet, F. B., (2001). Lassa fever in Guinea: I. Epidemiology of human disease and clinical observations. *Vector-Borne and Zoonotic Diseases, 1*(4), 269–281.

19. Benner, C., Carabin, H., Sánchez-Serrano, L. P., Budke, C. M., & Carmena, D., (2010). Analysis of the economic impact of cystic echinococcosis in Spain. *Bulletin of the World Health Organization, 88*, 49–57B.

20. Bergevoet, R. H. M., Van, S. G., Veling, J., Backus, G. B. C., & Franken, P., (2009). Economic and epidemiological evaluation of salmonella control in Dutch dairy herds. *Preventive Veterinary Medicine, 89*(1, 2), 1–7.

21. Binder, V., (1988). Epidemiology, course and socio-economic influence of inflammatory bowel disease. *Schweizerische Medizinische Wochenschrift (Swiss Medical Weekly), 118*(20), 738.

22. Bolos, B., Bacarea, V., & Marusteri, M., (2011). Approaching economic issues through epidemiology: An introduction to business epidemiology. *Romanian Journal of Economic Forecasting, 14*(1), 257–276.

23. Bonds, M. H., Keenan, D. C., Rohani, P., & Sachs, J. D., (2010). Poverty trap formed by the ecology of infectious diseases. *Proceedings of the Royal Society B: Biological Sciences, 277*(1685), 1185–1192.

24. Boni, M. F., Galvani, A. P., Wickelgren, A. L., & Malani, A., (2013). Economic epidemiology of avian influenza on smallholder poultry farms. *Theoretical Population Biology, 90*, 135–144.

25. Bonovas, S., & Nikolopoulos, G., (2012). High-burden epidemics in Greece in the era of economic crisis. Early signs of a public health tragedy. *Journal of Preventive Medicine and Hygiene, 53*(3).

26. Borghol, N., Suderman, M., McArdle, W., Racine, A., Hallett, M., Pembrey, M., & Szyf, M., (2012). Associations with early-life socio-economic position in adult DNA methylation. *International Journal of Epidemiology, 41*(1), 62–74.

27. Brandes, S. B., (2008). Epidemiology, etiology, histology, classification, and economic impact of urethral stricture disease. In: *Urethral*

Reconstructive Surgery (pp. 53–61). Humana Press.

28. Brown, M. L., Lipscomb, J., & Snyder, C., (2001). The burden of illness of cancer: Economic cost and quality of life. *Annual Review of Public Health, 22*(1), 91–113.
29. Buckley, C. H., (1984). A suggested remedy for toxic injury: Class actions, epidemiology, and economic efficiency. *Wm. and Mary L. Rev., 26*, 497.
30. Budke, C. M., Jiamin, Q. I. U., Qian, W., & Torgerson, P. R., (2005). Economic effects of echinococcosis in a disease-endemic region of the Tibetan Plateau. *The American Journal of Tropical Medicine and Hygiene, 73*(1), 2–10.
31. Bundy, D. A., Arámbulo, III. P. V., & Grey, C. L., (1983). Fascioliasis in Jamaica: Epidemiologic and economic aspects of a snail-borne parasitic zoonosis. *Bulletin of the Pan American Health Organization (PAHO), 17*(3), 1983.
32. Buzby, J. C., & Roberts, T., (2009). The economics of enteric infections: Human foodborne disease costs. *Gastroenterology, 136*(6), 1851–1862.
33. Bwire, G., Munier, A., Ouedraogo, I., Heyerdahl, L., Komakech, H., Kagirita, A., & Makumbi, I., (2017). Epidemiology of cholera outbreaks and socio-economic characteristics of the communities in the fishing villages of Uganda: 2011–2015. *PLoS Neglected Tropical Diseases, 11*(3), e0005407.
34. Canali, M., Aragrande, M., Angheben, A., Capelli, G., Drigo, M., Gobbi, F., & Cassini, R., (2020). Epidemiologic-economic models and the One Health paradigm: echinococcosis and leishmaniasis, case studies in Veneto region, Northeastern Italy. One Health, 9, 100115.
35. Casamassimo, P. S., Thikkurissy, S., Edelstein, B. L., & Maiorini, E., (2009). Beyond the DMFT: The human and economic cost of early childhood caries. *The Journal of the American Dental Association, 140*(6), 650–657.
36. Castro, M. C., Wilson, M. E., & Bloom, D. E., (2017). Disease and economic burdens of dengue. *The Lancet Infectious Diseases, 17*(3), e70–e78.
37. Chen, P. L., Li, C. Y., Hsieh, T. H., Chang, C. M., Lee, H. C., Lee, N. Y., & Ko, W. C., (2012). Epidemiology, disease spectrum and economic burden of non-typhoidal Salmonella infections in Taiwan, 2006–2008. *Epidemiology and Infection, 140*(12), 2256–2263.

38. Conover, M. R., Pitt, W. C., Kessler, K. K., DuBow, T. J., & Sanborn, W. A., (1995). Review of human injuries, illnesses, and economic losses caused by wildlife in the United States. *Wildlife Society Bulletin (1973–2006), 23*(3), 407–414.
39. Crump, J. A., Murdoch, D. R., & Baker, M. G., (2001). Emerging infectious diseases in an island ecosystem: The New Zealand perspective. *Emerging Infectious Diseases, 7*(5), 767.
40. Daily, G. C., & Ehrlich, P. R., (1996). Global change and human susceptibility to disease. *Annual Review of Energy and the Environment, 21*(1), 125–144.
41. Deogaonkar, R., Hutubessy, R., Van, D. P. I., Evers, S., & Jit, M., (2012). Systematic review of studies evaluating the broader economic impact of vaccination in low- and middle-income countries. *BMC Public Health, 12*(1), 878.
42. Dorn, C. R., (1992). Veterinary epidemiology and its economic importance in AD 2000. *Preventive Veterinary Medicine, 13*(2), 129–136.
43. Ducrotoy, M. J., Bertu, W. J., Ocholi, R. A., Gusi, A. M., Bryssinckx, W., Welburn, S., & Moriyon, I., (2014). Brucellosis as an emerging threat in developing economies: Lessons from Nigeria. *PLoS Negl. Trop. Dis., 8*(7), e3008.
44. Eaton, D. L., & Groopman, J. D., (2013). *The Toxicology of Aflatoxins: Human Health, Veterinary, and Agricultural Significance.* Elsevier.
45. Eckelman, M. J., Sherman, J. D., & MacNeill, A. J., (2018). Life cycle environmental emissions and health damages from the Canadian healthcare system: An economic-environmental-epidemiological analysis. *PLoS Medicine, 15*(7), e1002623.
46. Egger, G., (2011). Obesity, chronic disease, and economic growth: A case for "big picture" prevention. *Advances in Preventive Medicine*, 2011.
47. Elbe, S., (2007). Our epidemiological footprint: The circulation of avian flu, SARS, and HIV/AIDS in the world economy. *Review of International Political Economy, 15*(1), 116–130.
48. Ernst, R. L., & Hay, J. W., (1994). The US economic and social costs of Alzheimer's disease revisited. *American Journal of Public Health, 84*(8), 1261–1264.
49. Espinoza, J. R., Terashima, A., Herrera-Velit, P., & Marcos, L. A.,

(2010). Human and animal fascioliasis in Peru: Impact in the economy of endemic zones. *Revista Peruana de Medicina Experimental y Salud Publica (Peruvian Journal of Experimental Medicine and Public Health)*, 27(4), 604.

50. Ezzati, M., Vander, H. S., Lawes, C. M., Leach, R., James, W. P. T., Lopez, A. D., & Murray, C. J., (2005). Rethinking the "diseases of affluence" paradigm: Global patterns of nutritional risks in relation to economic development. *PLoS Med., 2*(5), e133.
51. Fenichel, E. P., (2013). Economic considerations for social distancing and behavioral based policies during an epidemic. *Journal of Health Economics, 32*(2), 440–451.
52. Fenichel, E. P., Castillo-Chavez, C., Ceddia, M. G., Chowell, G., Parra, P. A. G., Hickling, G. J., & Springborn, M., (2011). Adaptive human behavior in epidemiological models. *Proceedings of the National Academy of Sciences, 108*(15), 6306–6311.
53. Fogel, R. W., (1994). *Economic Growth, Population Theory, and Physiology: The Bearing of Long-Term Processes on the Making of Economic Policy (No. w4638)*. National Bureau of Economic Research.
54. Foxman, B., (2002). Epidemiology of urinary tract infections: Incidence, morbidity, and economic costs. *The American Journal of Medicine, 113*(1), 5–13.
55. Garner, M. G., Whan, I. F., Gard, G. P., & Phillips, D., (2001). The expected economic impact of selected exotic diseases on the pig industry of Australia. *Revue Scientifique et Technique-Office International des Epizooties (Plurithematic issue of the Scientific and Technical Review), 20*(3), 671–686.
56. Gayle, H. D., & Hill, G. L., (2001). Global impact of human immunodeficiency virus and AIDS. *Clinical Microbiology Reviews, 14*(2), 327–335.
57. Gottstein, B., Pozio, E., & Nöckler, K., (2009). Epidemiology, diagnosis, treatment, and control of trichinellosis. *Clinical Microbiology Reviews, 22*(1), 127–145.
58. Hart, O. E., & Halden, R. U., (2020). Computational analysis of SARS-CoV-2/COVID-19 surveillance by wastewater-based epidemiology locally and globally: Feasibility, economy, opportunities and challenges. *Science of The Total Environment*, 138875.
59. Häsler, B., Howe, K. S., & Stärk, K. D., (2011). Conceptualizing the

technical relationship of animal disease surveillance to intervention and mitigation as a basis for economic analysis. *BMC Health Services Research, 11*(1), 225.

60. Henschke, N., Kamper, S. J., & Maher, C. G., (2015). The epidemiology and economic consequences of pain. In: *Mayo Clinic Proceedings* (Vol. 90, No. 1, pp. 139–147). Elsevier.
61. Hochberg, M. C., (1992). Association of nonsteroidal anti-inflammatory drugs with upper gastrointestinal disease: Epidemiologic and economic considerations. *The Journal of Rheumatology and Supplement, 36*, 63–67.
62. Howe, K. S., Häsler, B., & Stärk, K. D. C., (2013). Economic principles for resource allocation decisions at the national level to mitigate the effects of disease in farm animal populations. *Epidemiology and Infection, 141*(1), 91–101.
63. Howe, L. D., Galobardes, B., Matijasevich, A., Gordon, D., Johnston, D., Onwujekwe, O., & Hargreaves, J. R., (2012). Measuring socio-economic position for epidemiological studies in low-and middle-income countries: A methods of measurement in epidemiology paper. *International Journal of Epidemiology, 41*(3), 871–886.
64. Jenkins, R., Baingana, F., Ahmad, R., McDaid, D., & Atun, R., (2011). Social, economic, human rights, and political challenges to global mental health. *Mental Health in Family Medicine, 8*(2), 87.
65. Johnson, R. W., Alvarez-Pasquin, M. J., Bijl, M., Franco, E., Gaillat, J., Clara, J. G., & Weinke, T., (2015). Herpes zoster epidemiology, management, and disease and economic burden in Europe: A multidisciplinary perspective. *Therapeutic Advances in Vaccines, 3*(4), 109–120.
66. Kim, J. J., & Goldie, S. J., (2008). Health and economic implications of HPV vaccination in the United States. *New England Journal of Medicine, 359*(8), 821–832.
67. Klein, E., Laxminarayan, R., Smith, D. L., & Gilligan, C. A., (2007). Economic incentives and mathematical models of disease. *Environment and Development Economics,* 707–732.
68. Klepac, P., Laxminarayan, R., & Grenfell, B. T., (2011). Synthesizing epidemiological and economic optima for control of immunizing infections. *Proceedings of the National Academy of Sciences, 108*(34), 14366–14370.

69. Krieger, N., (2001a). A glossary for social epidemiology. *Journal of Epidemiology and Community Health, 55*(10), 693–700.
70. Krieger, N., (2001b). Theories for social epidemiology in the 21st century: An eco-social perspective. *International Journal of Epidemiology, 30*(4), 668–677.
71. Lemma, A., (1969). Bilharziasis in the awash valley: I. An epidemiological study with special emphasis on its possible future economic and public health importance. *Ethiopian Medical Journal, 7*(4), 147–76.
72. Liu, J. L., Maniadakis, N., Gray, A., & Rayner, M., (2002). The economic burden of coronary heart disease in the UK. *Heart, 88*(6), 597–603.
73. López, N., Torné, A., Franco, A., San-Martin, M., Viayna, E., Barrull, C., & Perulero, N., (2018). Epidemiologic and economic burden of HPV diseases in Spain: Implication of additional 5 types from the 9-valent vaccine. *Infectious Agents and Cancer, 13*(1), 15.
74. Markos, T., & Abdela, N., (2016). Epidemiology and economic importance of pullorum disease in poultry: A review. *Global Veterinaria, 17*, 228–237.
75. Martin, D. P., & Shepherd, D. N., (2009). The epidemiology, economic impact and control of maize streak disease. *Food Security, 1*(3), 305–315.
76. McGuinness, D., McGlynn, L. M., Johnson, P. C., MacIntyre, A., Batty, G. D., Burns, H., & McGinty, A., (2012). Socio-economic status is associated with epigenetic differences in the pSoBid cohort. *International Journal of Epidemiology, 41*(1), 151–160.
77. Moné, H., Ibikounlé, M., Massougbodji, A., & Mouahid, G., (2010). Human schistosomiasis in the economic community of West African States: Epidemiology and control. In: *Advances in Parasitology* (Vol. 71, pp. 33–91). Academic Press.
78. Morand, O. F., (2004). Economic growth, longevity and the epidemiological transition. *The European Journal of Health Economics, Formerly: HEPAC, 5*(2), 166–174.
79. Moro, P. L., Budke, C. M., Schantz, P. M., Vasquez, J., Santivanez, S. J., & Villavicencio, J., (2011). Economic impact of cystic echinococcosis in Peru. *PLoS Negl. Trop. Dis., 5*(5), e1179.
80. Narrod, C., Zinsstag, J., & Tiongco, M., (2012). A one health framework

for estimating the economic costs of zoonotic diseases on society. *Eco Health, 9*(2), 150–162.

81. Nascimento, G. L., & De Oliveira, M. R. F., (2014). Severe forms of *Schistosomiasis mansoni*: Epidemiologic and economic impact in Brazil, 2010. *Transactions of the Royal Society of Tropical Medicine and Hygiene, 108*(1), 29–36.
82. O'Brien, J. A., Lahue, B. J., Caro, J. J., & Davidson, D. M., (2007). The emerging infectious challenge of Clostridium difficile-associated disease in Massachusetts hospitals: Clinical and economic consequences. *Infection Control and Hospital Epidemiology, 28*(11), 1219–1227.
83. Oleś, K., Gudowska-Nowak, E., & Kleczkowski, A., (2012). Understanding disease control: Influence of epidemiological and economic factors. *PloS One, 7*(5), e36026.
84. Otte, M. J., Nugent, R., & McLeod, A., (2004). *Transboundary Animal Diseases: Assessment of Socio-Economic Impacts and Institutional Responses* (pp. 119–126). Rome, Italy: Food and Agriculture Organization (FAO).
85. Ozawa, S., Portnoy, A., Getaneh, H., Clark, S., Knoll, M., Bishai, D., & Patwardhan, P. D., (2016). Modeling the economic burden of adult vaccine-preventable diseases in the United States. *Health Affairs, 35*(11), 2124–2132.
86. Ozmen, O., Kurşun, O., & Ozcelik, M., (2005). Bovine tuberculosis in Burdur, southern Turkey: Epidemiological, pathological and economic study. *The International Journal of Tuberculosis and Lung Disease, 9*(12), 1398–1402.
87. Paarlberg, P. L., Hillberg, A., Lee, J. G., & Mathews, Jr. K. H., (2008). *Economic Impacts of Foreign Animal Disease (No. 1477-2016-121206).*
88. Paisley, L. G., Vraa-Andersen, L., Dybkjaer, L., Møller, K., Christensen, G., Mousing, J., & Agger, J. F., (1993). An epidemiologic and economic study of respiratory diseases in two conventional danish swine herds. I: Prevalence of respiratory lesions at slaughter and their effects on growth. *Acta Veterinaria Scandinavica, 34*(4), 319–329.
89. Pal, M., Kerorsa, G. B., Marami, L. M., & Kandi, V., (2020). Epidemiology, pathogenicity, animal infections, antibiotic resistance, public health significance, and economic impact of Staphylococcus

aureus: A comprehensive review. *American Journal of Public Health, 8*(1), 14–21.

90. Paterson, A. D., Otte, M. J., Slingenbergh, J., Wint, W., & Rogers, D., (2000). The application of GIS and remote sensing-based modeling techniques, for use in the economic and epidemiological assessment of disease control interventions, at a regional or national level. In society for veterinary epidemiology and preventive medicine. *Proceedings of a Meeting Held at the University of Edinburgh on the 29th, 30th and 31st of March 2000* (pp. 172–182). Society for Veterinary Epidemiology and Preventive Medicine.
91. Pearce, N., & Merletti, F., (2006). Complexity, Simplicity, and Epidemiology. *International journal of epidemiology, 35*(3), 515-519.
92. Peckham, R., (2013). Economies of contagion: Financial crisis and pandemic. *Economy and Society, 42*(2), 226–248.
93. Perrings, C., Castillo-Chavez, C., Chowell, G., Daszak, P., Fenichel, E. P., Finnoff, D., & Levin, S., (2014). Merging economics and epidemiology to improve the prediction and management of infectious disease. *EcoHealth, 11*(4), 464–475.
94. Perrings, C., Williamson, M., Barbier, E. B., Delfino, D., Dalmazzone, S., Shogren, J., & Watkinson, A., (2002). Biological invasion risks and the public good: An economic perspective. *Conservation Ecology, 6*(1).
95. Perry, B. D., & Randolph, T. F., (1999). Improving the assessment of the economic impact of parasitic diseases and of their control in production animals. *Veterinary Parasitology, 84*(3, 4), 145–168.
96. Philipson, T. J., & Posner, R. A., (1996). The economic epidemiology of crime. *The Journal of Law and Economics, 39*(2), 405–433.
97. Philipson, T., (2000). Economic epidemiology and infectious diseases. *Handbook of Health Economics, 1*, 1761–1799.
98. Pongchaiyakul, C., Songpattanasilp, T., & Taechakraichana, N., (2008). Osteoporosis: Overview in disease, epidemiology, treatment and health economy. *Medical Journal of the Medical Association of Thailand, 91*(4), 581.
99. Poundstone, K. E., Strathdee, S. A., & Celentano, D. D., (2004). The social epidemiology of human immunodeficiency virus/acquired immunodeficiency syndrome. *Epidemiologic Reviews, 26*(1), 22–35.
100. Pritchett, J. G., Thilmany, D. D., & Johnson, K. K., (2005). Animal

disease economic impacts: A survey of literature and typology of research approaches. *International Food and Agribusiness Management Review, 8*(1030-2016-82471), 23–45.

101. Pugliatti, M., Beghi, E., Forsgren, L., Ekman, M., & Sobocki, P., (2007). Estimating the cost of epilepsy in Europe: A review with economic modeling. *Epilepsia, 48*(12), 2224–2233.

102. Purevdawa, E., Moon, T. D., Baigalmaa, C., Davaajav, K., Smith, M. L., & Vermund, S. H., (1997). Rise in sexually transmitted diseases during democratization and economic crisis in Mongolia. *International Journal of STD and AIDS, 8*(6), 398–401.

103. Ramesh, G. N., Malla, N., Raju, G. S., Sehgal, R., Ganguly, N. K., Mahajan, R. C., & Dilawari, J. B., (1990). Epidemiological study of parasitic infestations in lower socio-economic group in Chandigarh (North India). *Indian Journal of Medical Research. Section A, Infectious Diseases, 93,* 47–50.

104. Raut, L. K., (2004). *Economic Epidemiology of Malaria and Income Growth*. Available at: SSRN 832446.

105. Rehm, J., Mathers, C., Popova, S., Thavorncharoensap, M., Teerawattananon, Y., & Patra, J., (2009). Global burden of disease and injury and economic cost attributable to alcohol use and alcohol-use disorders. *The Lancet, 373*(9682), 2223–2233.

106. Rich, K. M., & Perry, B. D., (2011). The economic and poverty impacts of animal diseases in developing countries: New roles, new demands for economics and epidemiology. *Preventive Veterinary Medicine, 101*(3, 4), 133–147.

107. Rogers, J., Carolin, T., Vaught, J., & Compton, C., (2011). Biobankonomics: A taxonomy for evaluating the economic benefits of standardized centralized human biobanking for translational research. *Journal of the National Cancer Institute Monographs, 2011*(42), 32–38.

108. Ronohardjo, P., & Rastiko, P., (1982). Some epidemiological aspects and economic loss of bovine ephemeral fever outbreak in Tuban and surrounding areas, East Java, Indonesia. *Penyakit Hewan, 14*(24), 25–29.

109. Sachs, J., & Malaney, P., (2002). The economic and social burden of malaria. *Nature, 415*(6872), 680–685.

110. Sachs, J., (2001). *Macroeconomics and Health: Investing in Health for*

Economic Development. World Health Organization.

111. Saleha, A. A., (1991). Liver fluke disease (fascioliasis): Epidemiology, economic impact and public health significance. *Southeast Asian J. Trop. Med. Public Health, 22*(361), 4.
112. Sibert, L., Rigaud, J., Delavierre, D., & Labat, J. J., (2010). Chronic pelvic pain: Epidemiology and economic impact. *Progres En Urologie: Journal De L'association Francaise D'urologie Et De La Societe Francaise D'urologie (Progress in Urology: Journal of the French Urology Association and of the French Urology Society), 20*(12), 872–885.
113. Skrepnek, G. H., & Skrepnek, S. V., (2004). Epidemiology, clinical and economic burden, and natural history of chronic obstructive pulmonary disease and asthma. *Am. J. Manag. Care, 10*(5), S129–138.
114. Sloane, D., (2009). Cancer epidemiology in the United States: Racial, social, and economic factors. In: *Cancer Epidemiology* (pp. 65–83). Humana Press.
115. Sockett, P., (1993). Social and economic aspects of food-borne disease. *Food Policy, 18*(2), 110–119.
116. St. George, T. D., (1986). The epidemiology of bovine ephemeral fever in Australia and its economic effect. In Arbovirus research in Australia. *Proceedings Fourth symposium* (pp. 281–286). Brisbane, Australia. CSIRO.
117. Steben, M., & Duarte-Franco, E., (2007). Human papillomavirus infection: Epidemiology and pathophysiology. *Gynecologic Oncology, 107*(2), S2–S5.
118. Stehr-Green, J. K., & Schantz, P. M., (1987). The impact of zoonotic diseases transmitted by pets on human health and the economy. *Veterinary Clinics of North America: Small Animal Practice, 17*(1), 1–15.
119. Stuckler, D., & Siegel, K., (2011). *Sick Societies: Responding to the Global Challenge of Chronic Disease.* Oxford University Press.
120. Stuckler, D., (2008). Population causes and consequences of leading chronic diseases: A comparative analysis of prevailing explanations. *The Milbank Quarterly, 86*(2), 273–326.
121. Suhrcke, M., Stuckler, D., Suk, J. E., Desai, M., Senek, M., McKee, M., & Rechel, B., (2011). The impact of economic crises on communicable disease transmission and control: A systematic review of the evidence.

PloS One, 6(6), e20724.

122. Šumilo, D., Bormane, A., Asokliene, L., Vasilenko, V., Golovljova, I., Avsic-Zupanc, T., & Randolph, S. E., (2008). Socio-economic factors in the differential upsurge of tick-borne encephalitis in Central and Eastern Europe. *Reviews in Medical Virology, 18*(2), 81–95.

123. Tapia, G., (2003). Economics, demography, and epidemiology: An interdisciplinary glossary. *Journal of Epidemiology and Community Health, 57*(12), 929.

124. Torgerson, P. R., & Dowling, P. M., (2001). Estimating the economic effects of cystic echinococcosis. Part 2: An endemic region in the United Kingdom, a wealthy, industrialized economy. *Annals of Tropical Medicine and Parasitology, 95*(2), 177–185.

125. Torgerson, P. R., Carmona, C., & Bonifacino, R., (2000). Estimating the economic effects of cystic echinococcosis: Uruguay, a developing country with upper-middle-income. *Annals of Tropical Medicine and Parasitology, 94*(7), 703–713.

126. Uddin, K. S., Atanasova, K. R., Krueger, W. S., Ramirez, A., & Gray, G. C., (2013). Epidemiology, geographical distribution, and economic consequences of swine zoonoses: A narrative review. *Emerging Microbes and Infections, 2*(1), 1–11.

127. Uusküla, A., Müürsepp, A., Kawai, K., Raag, M., Jürisson, M., & Pillsbury, M., (2013). The epidemiological and economic impact of a quadrivalent human papillomavirus (HPV) vaccine in Estonia. *BMC Infectious Diseases, 13*(1), 304.

128. Vanni, T., Karnon, J., Madan, J., White, R. G., Edmunds, W. J., Foss, A. M., & Legood, R., (2011). Calibrating models in economic evaluation. *Pharmacoeconomics, 29*(1), 35–49.

129. Weycker, D., Edelsberg, J., Oster, G., & Tino, G., (2005). Prevalence and economic burden of bronchiectasis. *Clinical Pulmonary Medicine, 12*(4), 205–209.

130. Wu, T., Perrings, C., Kinzig, A., Collins, J. P., Minteer, B. A., & Daszak, P., (2017). Economic growth, urbanization, globalization, and the risks of emerging infectious diseases in China: A review. *Ambio, 46*(1), 18–29.

131. Yach, D., Stuckler, D., & Brownell, K. D., (2006). Epidemiologic and economic consequences of the global epidemics of obesity and diabetes. *Nature Medicine, 12*(1), 62–66.

132. Yi-Xin, H., & Manderson, L., (2005). The social and economic context and determinants of schistosomiasis japonica. *Acta Tropica, 96*(2, 3), 223–231.

133. Zadoks, J. C., (2008). *On the Political Economy of Plant Disease epidemicsDisease epidemics: Capita Selecta in Historical Epidemiology*. Wageningen Academic Publishers.

134. Zhan, P., Li, D., Wang, C., Sun, J., Geng, C., Xiong, Z., & De Hoog, G. S., (2015). Epidemiological changes in tinea capitis over the 60 years of economic growth in China. *Medical Mycology, 53*(7), 691–698.

135. Zhang, M., Song, Y., Cai, X., & Zhou, J., (2008). Economic assessment of the health effects related to particulate matter pollution in 111 Chinese cities by using economic burden of disease analysis. *Journal of Environmental Management, 88*(4), 947–954.

INDEX

D

E

F

O

P

R

S

T

U

V